A Comprehensive Handbook *of* TRADITIONAL CHINESE MEDICINE

Prevention & Natural Healing

By Zhang Yifang

Better Link Press

This book is edited and designed by the Editorial Committee of *Cultural China* series.

Text by Zhang Yifang
Tai Chi and Ba Duan Jin movement demonstration by Yu Chao
Photographs and computer graphics by Roger Yan, Wu Mengyue, Quanjing, PPBC, Getty Images
Menu design and photographs by Manuela Aldica
Cover and interior design by Wang Wei

Copy Editor: Shelly Bryant
Editor: Cao Yue
Editorial Director: Zhang Yicong

Senior Consultants: Sun Yong, Wu Ying, Yang Xinci
Managing Director and Publisher: Wang Youbu

ISBN: 978-1-60220-172-9

Address any comments about *A Comprehensive Handbook of Traditional Chinese Medicine: Prevention & Natural Healing* to:

Better Link Press
99 Park Ave
New York, NY 10016
USA

or

Shanghai Press and Publishing Development Co., Ltd.
F 7 Donghu Road, Shanghai, China (200031)
Email: comments_betterlinkpress@hotmail.com

Printed in China by Shanghai Donnelley Printing Co., Ltd.

1   3   5   7   9   10   8   6   4   2

Contents

Introduction 7

Part One
General Theory and Concepts: Decoding the Coded Message of Chinese Medicine 14

Chapter One   The Concept of TCM   16

Chapter Two   The Theory of Yin and Yang   20

Chapter Three   Using the Five Elements   27

Chapter Four   The System of Organs and Meridians   36

Chapter Five   The Material Foundation of the Body   51

Chapter Six   Knowing Our Constitution   60

Chapter Seven   Why Do We Become Sick   73

Chapter Eight   Catching Early Signals from Our Body   91

Part Two
TCM External Adjustment: The Mystery of Meridians and Acupoints 108

Chapter Nine   How Are Meridians Related to Our Health   110

Chapter Ten   Meridian Maps and Self-Adjustment Points   119

Chapter Eleven   Acupuncture   133

Chapter Twelve   Moxibustion and Related Warmth Therapies   140

Chapter Thirteen   Tuina Manipulation and Chinese Massage   147

Chapter Fourteen Cupping Therapy   153

Chapter Fifteen   Gua Sha Scraping Therapy   159

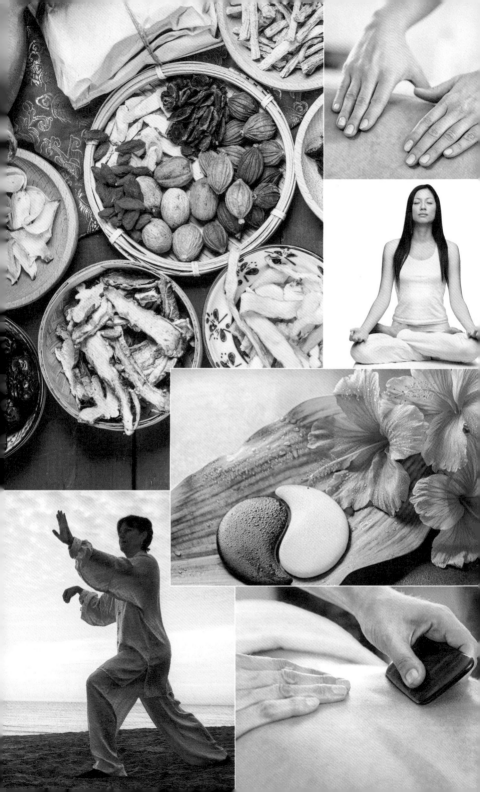

Part Three

TCM Internal Management: How Do Diet, Daily Lifestyle and Breath Control Affect Us 166

Chapter Sixteen   Functional Foods and Recipes   167

Chapter Seventeen   The Chinese Materia Medica and Prescriptions   184

Chapter Eighteen   Control of the Breath   207

Chapter Nineteen   Sleep and Meditation   214

Chapter Twenty   Tai Chi   223

Chapter Twenty-One   Ba Duan Jin   230

Chapter Twenty-Two   Healthy Lifestyle: Regulation of Daily and
                    Seasonal Rhythms, Life Stages and Space   237

Appendices 263

Basic Concepts of TCM Health Care Defined by the State
    Administration of Traditional Chinese Medicine   263

Glossary   264

The Top Six Groups of Healthy and Anti-Age Plants   269

Seasonal Foods   275

Three Case Studies in Longevity   276

The Categorization of Prescriptions According to the Specific
    Function of Chinese Medical Herbs   281

Self-Help Meridian Points and Their Locations   283

Comprehensive Methods for Preventing Influenza   287

Index   289

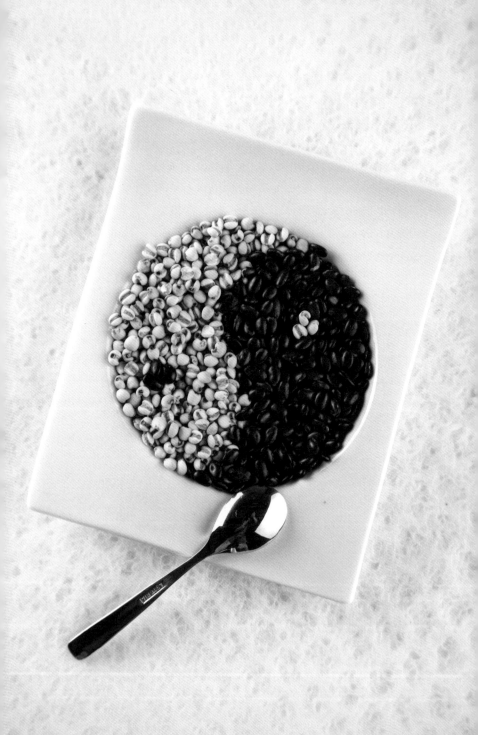

Introduction

We are what we read and think.
We are what we eat.
We are what we connect.
(Proverb)

"We are what we read and think" means the books we read enrich our experience and enhance our health awareness. Medical knowledge in the East and West is based on philosophical thinking, logical inference, and clinical examination. All medicine is the accumulation of human wisdom and experience. Understanding this body of knowledge will make one more objective, selective, and rational and will arm us with more solutions when we face health issues.

"We are what we eat" indicates that food shapes us. The diet we choose and the food we consume contribute to our unique body constitution. The healthy eating concepts and habits advocated in this book, combined with a wealth of anti-aging and preventive food and herbs, remedies, and recipes, will help us enjoy food while staying healthy.

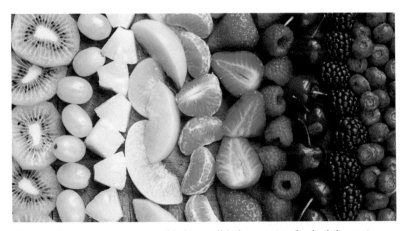

The healthy eating concepts and habits will help us enjoy food while staying healthy.

"We are what we connect" means our internal and external biospheres decide our lifespan. The internal and external network of relationships unifies the inside and outside of the human body. The body's internal network includes visible or invisible electric currents and magnetic conduction, the nervous system, the respiratory tract, the esophagus, the lymphatic vessels, the blood vessels, the interstitial fluid system, and other such systems. Two thousand five hundred years ago, TCM (Traditional Chinese Medicine) created and discovered the meridians and triple-energized system, a higher level of the body's interconnected network, viewed from the perspective that human body is an organic whole. Our external social circle includes our family, friends, and neighbors. When we are not well, who cares about us and how many people care about us are relevant to our health. Research shows that the importance of interpersonal relationship to our longevity is far beyond imagination. Relationships may be more important than how much fruits and vegetables we eat and whether we exercise regularly and do regular physical checkups. A follow-up study of 268 men by Harvard Medical School found that what really matters in a person's life is his or her relationship with others. The study also found that people who spend a lot of time with friends and chatting tend to live longer than those who prefer to be alone.[1]

Seeking wise, effective solutions to achieve daily happiness, high quality of life, and longevity has become increasingly popular among individuals and families internationally. Understanding the theory and concepts of TCM, applying acupuncture (or acupressure), and the use of natural foods and herbs, combined with Qigong exercises and other similar activities have become routinely practiced worldwide in over 180 countries and regions. TCM provides a systematic philosophy and choices for people to cope with high pressure from living, working, and studying and challenges from an unhealthy lifestyle, because TCM is based on a bulk of clinical practices, thousands years' of development, and modern knowledge. Its logic is based on the foundation of harmony between

---

[1] American psychology professors Howard Friedman and Leslie Martin, "Longevity Engineering", 2011.

environmental conditions, food, and the human spirit.

People are eager to find easy ways to maintain a positive attitude toward life, and seek a healthy diet, exercise, and so on. Among the solutions for achieving physical and spiritual health, daily health care and disease prevention are far more important than treatments after symptoms have occurred. Therefore, we should build up our sense of health consciousness, know our own and family members' conditions, embrace those health care methods, choose suitable types or tools for health practice, and benefit ourselves in the long run.

The health management proposed by TCM is set on the basis of a "return to nature." Focus shifts away from treatment and rehabilitation to a certain measure of mind-body or illness's holistic adjustment, prevention, and maintenance. This is the principle applied in this book. When seeking health and well-being, we should look for help from the wisdom and methods classical, modern, Asian, and Western. As for individual health, one should achieve physical and mental harmony through maintaining the balance between heaven, earth, and humans.

I grew up in a family of TCM doctors and have been practicing TCM for nearly four decades. I have always followed the ideas of balance and harmony. I will share with you my accumulated experience and techniques in this book. A considerable part of the book is drawn from lectures I have delivered to various audiences at home and abroad, so the reader need not have a modern medical foundation or any knowledge about Chinese medicine. A variety of readers can find essential relevant knowledge and information from this book. In view of this goal, the style of writing is as close as possible to the readers, so that it is easy to learn, understand, and operate. Some who have TCM knowledge and those who want to use it as textbook for training can also find useful information in relevant chapters.

The wisdom of Chinese medicine is rooted in daily life and has been tested for thousands of years. Mindset is often emphasized first when we talk about our daily regimen. Psychological effects can be thought of as one's attitude toward overall wellness and total health maintenance, sometimes called the Health Quotient (HQ). According to this belief, whenever doctors of Chinese medicine see a conflict between the patient's body, environment, certain foods, and/or climate, they do not immediately look for a prescriptive remedy. Instead, they first seek to discover the root of the conflict, then they take steps to avoid a continuation of this conflict. Finally, they use food therapy, acupuncture, and lifestyle change, among other treatments, especially natural remedies that aim to eliminate the conflict and balance the body. When people receive modern treatment, functional food, acupressure, Qigong exercise, and other treatments provide beneficial adjuvants to these treatments, bringing complementary benefits to these people.

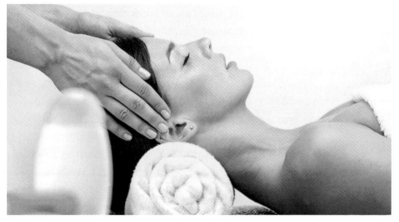

Use natural remedies to eliminate the conflict and balance the body.

Using food in a therapeutic way (which we term "functional foods" in this book), or adding external manipulation to the organ systems through the stimulation of meridians, channels and acupressure/acupuncture points, which are conduits for the flow of vital energy is a superior method of treating bodily disorders and preventing their recurrence. In addition, all therapy will have much better results when combined with healthy lifestyle practices, such as a positive view of life, getting enough sunlight, relaxation and sound sleep. Through these practices, we are forced to listen to our body, learn about ourselves, and gain a greater knowledge of what the body wants and needs.

Food therapy and acupuncture (or acupressure) is what I discuss first when teaching or consulted by patients. After evaluating a patient's condition, learning what disease they suffer from, and looking at their type, I tell them which foods they should avoid and suggest the best foods to add to their diet. They can also choose external meridian-related techniques, such as TCM massage, acupuncture, warm treatment, and cupping. After a while, many people benefit from this holistic approach. For some diseases, clients have to take prescription medicine, but I also try to combine or add non-medical therapies to reduce the quantity and duration of prescription drugs.

My mother, who is 92 years old, has suffered from Parkinson's disease for eight years. To deal with her perennial constipation, stiffness, and pain, I frequently use acupuncture, pressure points on the ears, and warm methods. If I'm not at home, my mother uses a tapping tool to tap her meridians and acupoints (mainly painful or uncomfortable points) herself. In this way, my mother only uses 25% to 50% of the painkillers taken by a typical Parkinson's disease patient.

TCM is effective for treating geriatric diseases, chronic diseases, and more challenging diseases. This is one of the greatest advantages of TCM. Fang Lipei, a medical advisor to the ex-president of the United States, said that Western medicine cannot cure some chronic diseases, but Chinese medicine can cure them well. He said that the application of TCM in the United States shows that after the intervention of TCM, the length of hospital stays has been halved and medical expenses have been cut in half. Some more difficult or complicated diseases cannot be relieved through modern medicine, but traditional Chinese medicine has solved these problems. Two years ago, my mother often had sudden losses of consciousness in the afternoon and evening. We immediately pressed her Shuigou acupoint (GV 26) and Shixuan acupoints (EX-UE 11) at fingertips. After several seconds, she woke up, very tired and exhausted. A 24-hour ECG showed that my mum's heart stopped nearly 10 times a day, for a maximum of 5.7 seconds. The modern hospital doctor suggested that a pacemaker should be installed. My mother did not agree, saying she would like to take Chinese herbal medicine instead. After taking a herbal prescription containing red ginseng, the fainting did not occur again.

The organization of this book's content is influenced by the law of the life cycle and the relevant health conditions written in the classical *Yellow Emperor's Internal Canon of Medicine* (in Chinese

Huangdi Neijing, the classic includes *The Spiritual Pivot*, in Chinese *Ling Shu* and *Basic Questions*, in Chinese *Su Wen*). The structure of this book consists of three parts. The first provides an overall introduction to the major principles of TCM theory. We follow the human life cycle as the main frame, briefly reviewing the philosophical thinking of Chinese medicine about life quality, a healthy lifestyle, illness prevention, and health care. This part starts with the introduction of the "balanced" approach of TCM, particularly the fundamental life system of Yin and Yang. It then brings in major concepts of the theory, the Five Elements, to explain relationship between internal and external body functions, the roles of organs, energy flows based on the meridians, Qi (vital energy), Blood, and Body Fluid. Having understood these TCM principles, one can judge his or her own body constitution and the reasons causing illness, as well as form plans for prevention that incorporate these principles.

Physical and spiritual health can be improved and maintained through adjustment of one's external or internal system. TCM applies natural therapies to achieve this goal, and it proposes many methods and tools that are easy to learn and use and can be mastered by anyone. There are two main ways to adjust health conditions through TCM: external and internal. The external means of health improvement are based on self-diagnosis, exploring and using key meridian points.

The second part of the book introduces the unique meridian theory of TCM, alongside various illness prevention and treatment techniques derived from this theory. It also covers different types of external therapies to manage health of mind and body, teaching popular and easy self-healing methods, including acupuncture, Tuina (massage) manipulation, cupping, scraping, and moxibustion.

The third part of the book provides solutions and recipes for preventing and treating many kinds of illness, which are also called internal therapy. The internal means of maintaining health is linked with food and spiritual practices. This part begins with a discussion on why and how diet, daily lifestyle, and breathing exercises affect our health. It provides categories of easily obtained functional foods and recipes and recommends taking them in different seasons, age groups, and body and mood states. Commonly used herbal remedies and prescriptions are also analyzed. Some popular exercises accompanying TCM are introduced in this part, including breath control, sleep and meditation, Tai Chi (a kind of traditional Chinese shadow boxing), and Ba Duan Jin (eight trigrams boxing). Readers who already have basic TCM knowledge may also find the comprehensive explanation of daily rhythms, self regulation in TCM theory and way, and life cultivation in four seasons, time of the day, and geographic locations to be of particular value. With these easy techniques, anyone can help themselves to improve physical fitness and mental relaxation, adjusting daily and periodical lifestyle, strengthening functions of internal organs, and boosting the body's healing power and rehabilitation functions.

The life cycle is a continuous process of inheritance and evolution, and it is a process of adapting to and regulating the environment. Therefore, this book provides many detailed approaches and skills for adapting to changing elements, such as the body and mind's reaction to the sun and the moon, water and earth, and seasons and temperature. In the process of the gestation and maturity of individual lives, it is necessary for people to deal with many undetermined factors and make corresponding choices, which forms the uniqueness of individual physique.

We live in an internationalized era, sharing various foods from overseas and having more opportunities to travel to other countries. This book tries to sort some internationally available foods into healthy categories. I hope that readers can apply the TCM knowledge gained from this context to select proper local foods to benefit their health.

I hope the clear theories and the simple, effective, practical techniques will put you on the right path to resolve the health issues in your daily life and help you discover effective therapies tailored to your personal health. After having acquired a fundamental knowledge of the approaches used in TCM through this book, you will be equipped to further explore health maintenance theories and skills on your own in the future. An old Chinese saying reminds us that "you can lead a horse to water but you can't make him drink." If we are to adjust and strengthen our bodies and minds, we must engage in active, continuous, and even lifelong practice. It is my hope that this TCM book will be a gift to you, your family, and your friends.

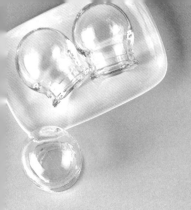

Part One

General Theory and Concepts: Decoding the Coded Message of Chinese Medicine

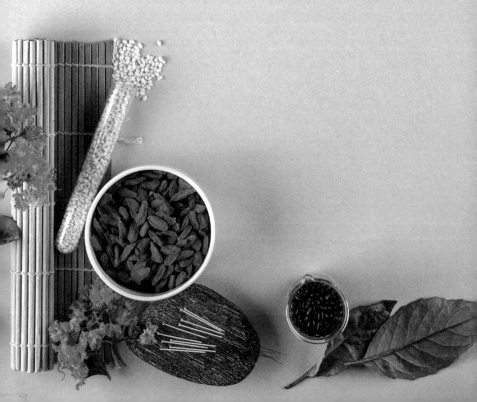

A Chinese proverb pointing to the inherent "correspondence between man and universe" indicates that relevant adaptation of the human body to its natural environment and society are key to keeping the human body healthy and constantly able to heal itself.

The food we eat, the pure water we drink, the clean air we breathe, the sunshine, the moonlight, and other natural forces form the strongest links between the universe and us. Maintaining a positive mental state, a healthy lifestyle, and personalized nutrition based on the individual's constitution are very important in TCM, but equally important is a holistic approach. A holistic approach means TCM focuses on the organic whole of the person, physiologically and psychologically, from head to toe, to bring the individual in balance with nature and society. It emphasizes using natural remedies (food, herbs, etc.), meridian-related therapy (acupressure, Tuina massage, acupuncture, cupping, Qigong exercise, etc.), and adjusting the mind before treating a condition with medicine. This approach helps us find the root cause of the unbalance, rather than just focusing on the symptoms. As the old saying goes, an ounce of prevention is worth a pound of cure. The preventative side of TCM provides an appealing, accessible point of entry for anyone who wants to learn about and use Chinese medicine. Food therapy and acupressure are the easiest ways to begin. Using plants and foods, self-exercise for health and the prevention of illness is deeply ingrained in China's rich culture.

Preventive health care has three aspects. The first is to keep us at a healthy level of fitness and enjoy ourselves more. This holistic approach is where freedom of body, mind, emotions and spirit flows.

The second aspect is to slow down the process of physical and psychological aging and strive for a longer and healthier life.

For the third aspect, genetic bias may kick in if we have a family history. Therefore, preventive health care can lessen or slow the onset of risks from a familial or hereditary diseases.

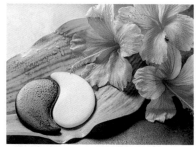

TCM emphasizes using natural healing.

Chapter One
The Concept of TCM

TCM has a history of 5,000 years. People have been solidifying TCM theory and technologies based on practical experience in human activities. It is a medical form originated from the Chinese Han ethnic group. (There are 56 ethnic groups in China. The Han group is one of them, accounting around 91~92% of the total population. Mandarin is the language of the Han ethnic group.)

TCM is a style of traditional medicine that has a complete theoretical system, including various forms of herbal medicine, acupuncture and moxibustion, Tuina (massage), Qigong (exercise), and dietary therapy. It is widely used in China, and has begun gaining global recognition. It is a comprehensive medical system that studies human physiology and pathology, disease diagnosis, prevention, and treatment, as well as health care and rehabilitation.

One of the basic tenets of TCM is that the body's vital energy (*chi* or Qi) circulates through channels, which are called "meridians," that have branches connected to bodily organs and functions. The concepts of the body and of its function as used in TCM reflect its ancient origins and its emphasis on dynamic processes over material structure, similar to European humoral theory.

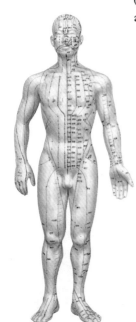

Meridians on human body.

What Are the Characteristics of TCM

The three fundamental characteristics of the TCM theory system are:

• A holistic concept based on the unique individual, centered on five organ systems connected by meridians. It gives attention to the person rather than the illness.

• Prevention and treatment plans are mainly based upon constitution types and identification of the disease syndromes.

• There is a correlation between man and nature. Nature refers to the seasonal changes, geographic location difference, and the variation of cultural and social environments. Our body is the corresponding system model between the inside and outside of the body, between heart and soul.

Let's take the second characteristic as an example. How do we define "constitution"? In daily practice, our body type is divided into Cold, Hot, Damp, and Dry. Syndrome differentiation includes summarizing and analyzing the clinical data of symptoms and signs collected with the four diagnostic methods (namely looking, listening and smelling, asking, and feeling) and categorizing it as a type of syndrome.

A syndrome is called *zheng* 证 in Chinese, which is a summary of the pathological changes of a disease at a certain stage in its course of development, including the location, cause, and nature of the disease, as well as the state of the relationship between *xie* 邪 (pathogenic factors) and *zheng* 正 (the healthy Qi). The strategy is established accordingly, followed by methods of treatment, prescription of herbs or acupuncture points, or Tuina procedures. TCM doctors will inform you of the frequency and duration of the medical treatment that ought to be followed, combined with some diet and lifestyle changes for prevention.

Take the flu as an example. Modern vaccines against influenza are the same for everyone when they suffer from the flu. The main treatments are also similar for everyone. Treating the flu through TCM, the TCM doctor will identify 3 to 4 clinical types. The method of treatment will follow these types. This is because different human bodies with the same virus will exhibit very different clinical syndromes. Therefore, the method of treatment will be different, followed by an individualized diet and more physical exercise.

In 1956, when encephalitis B broke out, TCM doctor Pu Fuzhou treated 167 patients with encephalitis B, leading to no deaths. The 167 patients used 98 Chinese medicine prescriptions. On average, each prescription was used on two people or less. So we can see how TCM treats the same disease with different methods.

Western medicine has also learned from these ideas. A doctor does precise adjustments regarding the administration of medicine within the prescribed time, quantity, whether it can be combined with other medicines, and so forth. TCM doctors try to learn your disease first through Western medicine, then see your syndromes, which display a combination of the cause of illness and the reaction of the human body.

What Are the Advantages of TCM

Health status can be divided into: health cultivation, clinical symptoms, disease, serious disease, and surgery. For the first three items, advancement in TCM have provided many methods and tools to improve and restore health, which allow the two latter conditions to be better integrated with modern medicine and new technology.

Modern medicine and TCM use different methods, study, and research to study the human body from different angles. Each has its own advantages.

TCM, especially acupuncture, has thrived and flourished throughout the world, even blossoming deep in the medical systems of other locales around the world. Another application of acupuncture, called "dry needles," has been very popular in the US. Tai Chi and Ba Duan Jin exercise have been recognized and actively used by many countries around the world to relieve pain and stress. TCM has made a profound impact on human health maintenance and made great contributions to disease recovery.

Compared with modern medicine, which uses anatomical and experimental methods to look at human functions and judge health or disease, TCM studies the human body more macroscopically, and puts it into consideration in the natural environment, emphasizing the trinity of heaven, earth, and humans. The human system is like a little universe, and many of the laws and movement of the universe can be used to guide and inspire people's thinking on the path to health and the balance between the dynamic and the static.

China has 5,000 years of civilization. Chinese philosophy and medical experience and the written records related to Chinese medicine can be traced back about 3,000 years. The experience of health care and disease treatment accumulated over earlier periods has great application, and some experiences are clinical repeatable. It is reproducible and can be used by other disciplines. TCM is the common heritage of mankind and has gradually spread to all parts of the world. According to the 2018 literature of the State Administration of TCM, acupuncture and herbal medical practices have been applied in 183 countries and regions around the world, which fully proves that the universal effectiveness of TCM for humans is not limited to Chinese people or culture.

For chronic diseases, such as cancer, atrophic gastritis, eczema, allergic diseases, female hormonal syndrome, anxiety disorders, and ulcerative colitis, whose causes and pathological mechanisms cannot be explained by modern medicine, TCM can provide different perspectives and explanations, offering effective personal solutions to restore countless people's health.

Health Quotient

The ability and knowledge to control your own health can be called a high health quotient. It can be simply summarized as a good moral quality, clear health awareness, correct health knowledge, self-implementation of a healthy lifestyle initiative, and continuous execution. Health awareness is the key. The following 10 questions can help assess your sense of health consciousness.

1. Do you watch (or listen to, read) health information programs on media, books, or from TV?
☐(1) Never ☐(2) Occasionally
☐(3) Often ☐(4) Always

2. Can you make the right distinction between unclear health information and recognition?
☐(1) Unable ☐(2) Occasionally
☐(3) Often ☐(4) Always

3. Are you aware of your health problems?
☐(1) Never ☐(2) Occasionally
☐(3) Frequently ☐(4) Always

4. Do you realize that you should change your lifestyle for your health?
☐(1) No ☐(2) Occasionally
☐(3) Recently realized ☐(4) I'm aware of that

5. You think your health should be
☐(1) Whatever ☐(2) Based on luck
☐(3) Cared by doctors ☐(4) In my own hands

6. Which of the following priorities do you think best represents your opinion?

☐(1) Make money first ☐(2) Success comes first
☐(3) The quality of life comes first ☐(4) Health first

7. Do you know which lifestyle is not good for health and which is good for health?

☐(1) Never cared ☐(2) Know something
☐(3) Basic understanding ☐(4) Very clear

8. Do you know what your greatest health hazard is?

☐(1) I didn't think about it ☐(2) Sometimes I think about it
☐(3) Basically understand ☐(4) Very clear

9. Do you care about your mental health?

☐(1) Never ☐(2) Occasional
☐(3) Often ☐(4) Always

10. Do you buy health insurance?

☐(1) Never bought it ☐(2) Only bought it once or twice
☐(3) I did, but I never used it ☐(4) Always buy and use it

Assessment:
(1) 0 (2) 1 (3) 2 (4) 3

The scores of these 10 questions are totally 30 points, 18 points is passing, and the higher points the better. From answering above 10 questions you can have a preliminary assessment of your health awareness.

Chapter Two
The Theory of Yin and Yang

Dr. Gan Zuwang, who was one of my teachers, lived to the age of 103. He was a great master of TCM. When he was summarizing the secrets of keeping himself young minded and living a long and healthy life, he used a four-word proverb: *gui yu hou xing*, which means lowering desire like a turtle and gaining agility like a monkey. The turtle is slower to desire, avoiding conflict and making less trouble for others. It does not act on impulse, but always makes concessions and conquers the unyielding with the yielding. The monkey, as a quick thinker, reacts to things promptly and is very active and always full of energy.

Some of turtle's and monkey's habits are worth learning and emulating.

The turtle has a long lifespan. It can live a thousand years, and sometimes up to ten thousand years. The words *gui yu* (less desire, like a turtle) emphasizes that in the pursuit of a healthy body and a long life, it is necessary to reduce desire and maintain a quiet state of mind.

As in farming, people not only harvest in the autumn, but also remain in "hibernation" in the winter. All these points are the static part of a person, what is called Yin.

Monkeys are smart, naughty, and funny, and they own a much more highly developed brain. In the famous piece of work *The Journey to the West*, the Monkey King (Sun Wukong) was born intelligent, lively, and loyal, and he became an example of wit and bravery in Chinese culture, which represents hospitality, uprightness, being outspoken, and the pursuit of freedom and compassion in human nature. An "agile thinker, like a monkey" expresses openness of thought and the constant movement of the body, which allows the body and soul to be full of vitality. Both are circulated and dynamic, and are called Yang. Such a balanced and harmonized state of Yin and Yang can ensure a higher state of health.

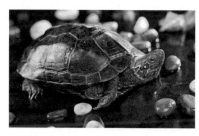
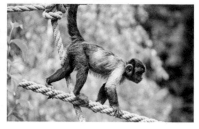

Lowering desire like a turtle.

Gaining agility like a monkey.

Origin and Principles of Yin and Yang

The Yin and Yang is an ancient philosophical concept which is at the core of TCM. The Yin and Yang are two fundamental principles

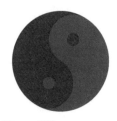

Yin and Yang.

or forces in the universe, constantly opposing and supplementing each other. All things and phenomena in the natural world contain the two opposing components of Yin and Yang. Examples include the sky and earth, heat and cold, or active and static states.

Here, we should take a step back for a moment and explore the basic concepts of Yin and Yang more thoroughly. In the beginning, Yin and Yang described a physical or geographical location in relation to the sun. The places exposed to the sun are Yang, and a place without exposure is Yin. The southern side of a mountain, for example, is Yang, while its northern side is Yin. Thus, the ancient Chinese people, in the course of their everyday lives and work, came to understand that all aspects of the natural world could be seen as having dual aspects. For example, day and night, brightness and dimness, movement and stillness, and upwards and downwards all express the Yin-Yang dichotomy.

The terms Yin and Yang are applied to express these dual and opposite qualities. Chapter Six of the ancient TCM classic *Basic Questions* states that "water and fire are symbols of Yin and Yang," so we can remember the features of Yin and Yang by comparing them with water and fire, or things that embodies similarly opposite characteristics, such as the sun and moon.

The content of the theory of Yin and Yang can be described briefly as opposition, interdependence, relative waxing and waning, and transformation.

1. Opposition and Interdependence of Yin and Yang

By the opposition of Yin and Yang, we mean that all things and phenomena in the natural world contains two opposite components: heaven and earth, outside and inside, movement and stability, and so forth. In the theory of Yin and Yang, heaven is considered Yang, while earth is Yin; outside is Yang, while inside is Yin; and movement is Yang, while stability is Yin.

Yin and Yang are not only opposite but also embody each other. Neither could exist without the other component. For instance, without outside, there would be no inside, and vice versa. This relationship of coexistence is known as interdependence. TCM holds that "functional movement" belongs to Yang and "nourishing substance" to Yin, and that the one cannot exist without the other.

2. The Waxing and Waning of Yin and Yang and the Transformation between Yin and Yang

Yin and Yang are not stagnant, but exist in a dynamic state. While Yin wanes, Yang waxes, and vice versa. This dynamic change of succession is known as the waxing and waning of Yin and Yang. Take the seasonal climatic variation in the natural world for example. The weather gets warm when winter gives way to spring, and becomes hot when spring gives way to summer, during which time Yin wanes while Yang waxes. However, it gets cool when autumn replaces summer and cold when winter replaces autumn, during which time Yang wanes but Yin waxes.

By "transformation," we mean Yin and Yang will transform into one another under certain conditions. For instance, in the course of suffering from a disease, a patient may run a high fever, have a red complexion, feel irritable and restless, and have a rapid and strong pulse, indicating strong Yang. Then, sometimes quite suddenly, he may show Yin characteristics, feeling listless with a low temperature, pale face, and weak pulse. This is an example of transformation from Yang to Yin.

How Do Yin and Yang Influence You Positively

• Knowing yourself and foods better will allow you to eat well.

• Always think of the golden mean (middle course between extremes) and balance of your body and soul (physical and mental functions).

• Choose your prevention, anti-aging, and longevity lifestyle and methods more easily.

Yin-Yang Theory—Achieving Balance: Harmonizing Quietness and Action

In Yin-Yang theory, the concept of opposites is key. For prevention and good health, Yin needs to be balanced with Yang, that is to say, action needs to be balanced with quietness.

To build Yin energy, everyone needs quiet time. The frequency depends on the individual and their personality. It can be achieved through spending time alone to recharge, getting adequate sleep, and resting, physically and mentally, or through activities such as meditation, massage, breathing techniques, and acupuncture. People with active jobs who spend time interacting with people and moving around all day should focus on finding quietness.

Building Yang energy requires action. The type of action depends on body constitution, character, and age group. It can be achieved through being physically active, taking part in sports, going to the gym, aerobic activity, swimming, dancing, and martial arts such as Tai Chi. People with sedentary jobs and little daily human interaction should focus on increasing action.

Controlling your breathing can influence overall energy and help your whole system to work together better as the kidney interacts with the lungs. Mindful breathing is a powerful way to reduce stress and combat sickness in today's busy world. Breathing in and out ensures energy flow into and out of the body. If we consciously breathe and bring energy deep into the body, we can keep energy levels high. Sometimes, during quiet moments, it is even possible to enter into a state of flow and subconsciousness.

It is essential to incorporate both action, for the physical body, and quiet, for the mind. If you combine the two, you will have a better quality of life and increase longevity.

Uses of Yin-Yang Theory in TCM

The Yin-Yang theory has been integral to the science of TCM, and its basic principals have played an important role in the formation and development of TCM's own theoretical system. It is used to explain tissue, structure, physiological functions, and pathological changes in the human body and to direct clinical diagnosis and treatment. It also forms a basis for the clinical application of Chinese food, medicinal herbs, and meridians. By doing so, one can achieve the goal of curing diseases.

1. The Yin-Yang Theory and the Movement of Qi

To achieve its function, the body's energy must maintain endless motion inside the body. If the movement slows down or runs in the wrong directions, one will suffer from illness. The movement of Qi has four directions: up, down, in, and out. The energy that goes up and out belongs to Yang action, while the energy that goes in and down belongs to Yin action. Energy movement is the basic form of Qi transformation in the human body, which triggers various changes and keeps organ function running smoothly. It is also the basic process to keep a harmonious relationship between viscera and the meridians. Therefore, the physiological function of organs and the meridians of the human body are dependent on the balance of energy's rise and fall, in and out. Examples are the energy of the lungs' disposal and descent, the spleen's ascending lucidity and the stomach's descending turbidity, the heart's fire and the kidney's water crossing each other, which are all specific embodiments of the movement of Qi. In the prevention of disease, it is also necessary to keep the human body's energy movements going up and down, in and out in a normal way, in order to resist invasion of toxins and avoid disease.

2. The Yin-Yang Theory and the Identification of the Ailment

When a patient visits a TCM clinic, the doctor will seek to understand the patient's symptoms according to the Yin-Yang theory. For example, when categorizing the characteristics of the face, tongue, and bodily excretions, the colors red, yellow, and green belong to Yang, while white and gray belong to Yin. A diagnosis is established based on the predominance or weakness of Yin and Yang. The Yin-Yang theory guides clinical treatments, such as the utilization of foods and herbs or the application of acupuncture according to one's property of Yin or Yang. A basic summary of this process is in the box below.

Clinical Processes of Using the Yin and Yang Theory

Case One

Symptoms: cold limbs, pale face, tongue that is pale with a white coating, affinity for hot drinks

TCM diagnosis: Yin pattern

Remedy: consume food and herbs with Yang characteristics, tapping or massage Yang meridian points

Case Two

Symptoms: sensation of burning or heat in the body, red face, red tongue with yellow coating, affinity for cold or iced drinks

TCM diagnosis: Yang pattern

Remedy: consume food and herbs with Yin characteristics, tapping or massage Yin meridian points

---

All the health care awareness and methods created from TCM are guided by the Yin and Yang, the balance between action and repose, work and rest, the reducing method and the reinforcing method. We must identify the Yin-Yang type of a person or his condition before practicing food therapy or increasing heat or cold treatments of external therapy.

3. The Yin-Yang Theory and the Application to Food

In TCM, Yin and Yang properties can be assigned to one's constitution as well as the food and herbs one consumes. A Yang constitution includes Hot, Dry, and overly strong properties of different body systems, while a Yin constitution demonstrates Cold, Damp, and weak properties. Yin foods, such as watermelon and mung bean, can bring nourishment and moisture internally, as well as to the skin and seven orifices. They can reduce Heat and calm the mind. Yang foods, such as walnut and cinnamon, can warm and energize the body, dry Dampness, and stimulate metabolism. Neutral foods, such as mushrooms, provide nutrition without influencing body systems. TCM uses foods to balance constitutions. For example, if a person's constitution has too much Yin, it can be neutralized by Yang food, and vice versa.

Let's examine what we mean by Yang and Yin foods and herbs. Yang means the metabolic temperature of the food is warm or hot. This is an inherent property and not necessarily dependent on the surface temperature of the food. Yang foods are more likely to be seasonal foods found in the winter. Things like root vegetables (parsnips, squash, mustard, and burdock) are excellent foods for warming and grounding us during the colder months. Cooking or

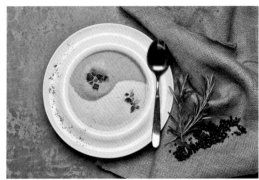

TCM uses foods to balance constitutions.

preparation methods include stir-frying, stewing, baking, deep-frying, roasting, grilling, and barbecuing. These foods and herbs make our body energy rise and come to the surface. Yin means the metabolic temperature of the food is cool or cold, and the taste is sour, bitter, or salty. These foods are found most plentifully in the summer, and are often eaten raw or steamed. Yin foods restrain our body's energy or cause it to descend. Some examples include sprouts, asparagus, grapefruit, avocado, and leafy green vegetables.

There are also many foods that have very mild Yin or Yang qualities, and therefore belong to the Neutral food category. Examples include rice, corn, beetroots, Chinese yams, kale, and carrots. Even if you do not have detailed knowledge about the Yin and Yang of food, you can quite naturally get a balance of Yin and Yang by consuming a broad range of foods and ensuring variety.

Our body's main 12 meridians are also divided into 6 Yang meridians and 6 Yin meridians, allowing us to choose to harmonize the Yin-Yang state. In times of illness or imbalance, learning about and applying food therapy, acupressure, and Qigong exercises will help you nourish your organs and strengthen your Yin-Yang energy.

Chapter Three
Using the Five Elements

In China's Jin dynasty (265–420), the famous doctor Zhang Zihe once treated a patient whose father was killed by a thief. Sorrow and tears caused him chest pressure and heartache, with the symptoms increasing over time, becoming worse. He reached out to the most famous doctors for medical treatment and accepted all kinds of drug formulas, but he gained nothing. When Dr. Zhang met the client, he happened to run into a witch at the patient's home. Inspired by the witch's ways, he combined various weird and funny physical gestures to make fun of the witch, which humored the patient and made him laugh. Two days later, his chest pressure and heartache were alleviated without the use of medicine.

How did happiness remedy his chest pressure and the heartache that occurred due to his excessive sadness?

According to the Five Elements Theory, happy feelings belong to the fire element, while sadness belongs to metal. In the natural world, fire can disperse and flare up. It melts metal materials such as gold. Increasing joyful moods (fire) can control sadness (metal). Sadness makes energy stagnant and blocked inside, so by finding a way to cheer a person up, the blocked Qi can be reopened and cleansed from the body. This summarizes the TCM psychological theory in relation to the five elements.

The universal goal everyone seeks is to achieve well-being. In our daily life, amid excessively lost, stressful conditions, it's advisable to think about joyful things and participate in group activities to help you relax. Activities such as singing, dancing, watching movies, going to operas, or traveling to great rivers and mountains can help eliminate worry and sadness. In Shanghai, there is a choir that gathers and sings every Sunday at Lu Xun Park. Many people with depression or sadness participate in the chorus, and they are gradually able to get rid of the medicine and restart their lives.

It's understandable that laughter, optimism, cheerfulness, less worries, and not hiding sad memories and feelings allow people to live happier and healthier lives.

The Formation of the Five Elements Theory

Each of the five elements has its special properties. This is also taken as one of the ancient philosophical concepts used in TCM.

Ancient philosophers made generalizations and deductions about the respective properties of the five kinds of substances and their relationships, in an effort to explain the entire material world. According to the theory of the five elements, wood, fire, earth, metal, and water are the five basic substances that constitute the material world. These substances are not only related through generation and restriction, but are also in a state of constant movement and change.

The Theory of the Five Elements

In Chinese, the five elements are called the *wu xing*. *Wu* means five and *xing* means movement and change. Each of the five elements— wood, fire, earth, metal, and water—have their own specific properties, but they also play interactive functions of generation and restriction. For example, earth generates metal but controls water, while earth, in turn, is restricted by wood. This means that the relationship between the elements is one of constant motion and change, each helping the others to stay relative equilibrium.

Together, the concepts of Yin-Yang and the five elements form the basis of traditional Chinese medical theory. They help explain the structures, functions, and relationships of different parts of the body and guide clinical diagnosis and treatment. The use of five elements in our daily life are mainly shown in three aspects:

- Understanding how our system can corporate with nature.
- Guiding us to understand the relationship between the internal organs.
- Guiding us to choose foods with different colors and flavors.

Life is like a five-flavored bottle. When we are born, the bottle is immediately overturned, and sour, sweet, bitter, spicy, and salty flavors fill the bottle one after another. When we are young, we already know that tears are salty, lemon is very sour, and herbs are quite bitter. Only after one has tasted bitter, salty, and sour, can he/she cherish the sweetness.

The therapeutic use of food in TCM is partially based on the five elements model, as each food or herb has a certain color and taste related to one of the elements. By determining a food's color, the color of the pulp is considered more than the pericarp.

The taste of a food or herb is not always related to its literal flavor. For instance, broccoli is classified as bitter and millet as salty. Taste, therefore, relates more to an intrinsic quality, rather than its literal flavor, although in most cases the two will coincide.

Clinically, Sour and Bitter tastes can be harmonized over sweet intakes or have the ability to control sugar cravings. Sweet is the taste of earth, while Sour and Bitter are the flavor of wood and fire, which restrict and generate the organ energy to reduce sweet intake.

Before exploring more about taste and flavor, we will first look at how the five elements theory is used to classify various things in nature, including the human body.

The Relationship between the Five Elements

Among the five elements, the main relation is based on generation and restriction.

Generation implies production and promotion. The order

of generation is wood generates fire, fire generates earth, earth generates metal, metal generates water, and water generates wood.

The relationship of generation of each of the five elements is composed of two aspects: generating and being generated. The element that generates is called the mother, while the element that is generated is called the son. Hence, the relation of generating and being generated among the five elements is also known as that of mother and son. Take wood for example, because wood produces fire, it is called the mother of fire. On the other hand, wood is produced by water, so it is called the son of water.

Restriction connotes bringing under control or restraint. The relationship of restriction between the five elements possess is that wood restricts earth, earth restricts water, water restricts fire, fire restricts metal, and metal restricts wood.

Each of the five elements plays the role of restricting and being restricted. Take wood for example. The element restricting wood is

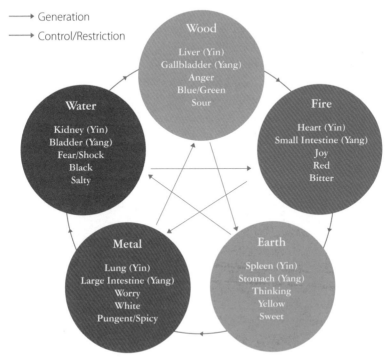

Relationship between the five elements.

metal, and the element that is restricted by wood is earth.

In view of the correlations among things in the material world, both generation and restriction are indispensable. Without generation, there would be no birth and development, but without restriction, excessive growth would result in harm. For instance, on one hand, wood generates fire, and on the other, it restricts earth, while earth, in its turn, generates metal and restricts water. Thus in generation there resides restriction, and in restriction there is generation. They oppose each other and at the same time cooperate with each other, maintaining a relative balance between generation and restriction and ensuring the normal growth and development of things.

The Content of the Five Elements: The Law of the Five Elements Connecting the Human Body and Nature

Based on the Five Elements Theory, TCM has conducted a comprehensive study of all things in nature and attributed each item to one of the five elements in accordance with its different properties, functions, and forms. This approach to understanding the physiology and pathology of the human body makes a strong correlation between humans and their natural surroundings. The tables below demonstrate how things are classified according to the five elements theory (more information about *zang* and *fu* organs can be found in the later section about internal organs).

The Five Elements and the Human Body						
Elements	*Zang* Organs	*Fu* Organs	Sense Organs	Tissue	Emotion	External Expression
Wood	Liver	Gallbladder	Eye	Tendons	Anger	Nail
Fire	Heart	Small intestine	Tongue	Vessels	Joy	Face
Earth	Spleen	Stomach	Mouth	Muscles	Thinking	Lip
Metal	Lung	Large intestine	Nose	Skin	Worry	Body hair
Water	Kidney	Bladder	Ear, lower orifices	Bone	Fear	Hair

Relationship between five elements and the human body.

			The Five Elements and the Nature				
Elements	Seasons	Environmental Factors	Growth & Development	Colors	Tastes	Orientation
Wood	Spring	Wind	Germination	Blue, green	Sour	East
Fire	Summer	Heat	Growth	Red	Bitter	South
Earth	Last 18 days of each season, rainy season	Dampness	Transformation	Yellow	Sweet	Middle
Metal	Autumn	Dryness	Reaping	White	Pungent (spicy)	West
Water	Winter	Coldness	Storing	Black	Salty	North

Relationship between five elements and the nature.

The following picture demonstrates a more comprehensive classification of things according to the five elements theory.

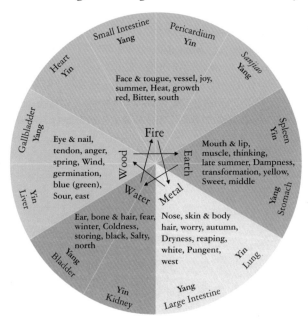

Classification of things according to the Five Elements Theory.

Applying the Five Elements in Food Therapy

The color and taste of food indicate an essential quality in that food, describing a potential that is liberated by the alchemy of cooking and digestion. As seen in the tables in the previous section on pages 31–32, the five elements theory holds that different colors of foods or herbs correspond with different organ systems and seasons. Each color and flavor arises from one elemental power and is said to enter a particular meridian and organ.

1. Food Colors

The Chinese phrase *"qing shan lu shui* 青山绿水 " refers to the turquoise mountain and water under the sunlight, a powerful metaphor for the landscape. Green improves vision and relaxes the mind. It further describes the deeper meaning that when we see those colors, it can cheer us up, open up our mind, and calm us down. The leaves and green mountains bring positive energy to us.

Green food corresponds with the liver system. Green foods are best for spring. They can regulate liver Qi and help the liver dispel toxins from the body. Too much alcohol and rich protein can harm the liver. There is a high relapse rate for liver ailments, especially chronic ones. Green foods are usually rich in fiber, vitamins, and chlorophyll, which help cleanse toxins.

The Chinese phrase *"bi xue dan xin* 碧血丹心 " means righteous blood and loyal heart (*dan xin* also literally means red heart). This idiom shows that red is matched to blood and the heart in Chinese culture.

Red food corresponds with the heart system. Red foods are best for summer. They help nourish blood, improve circulation, and reinforce Yang (warm) energy. They are usually recommended for people with anemia, palpitations, cold limbs, paleness, and weakness.

Yellow reminds us of rich soil and one of the earth colors, and "earth is mother of rest elements." It corresponds with the spleen system (digestive system), assists digestion, and helps reinforce spleen energy. Yellow foods are suitable year-round, but are particularly good for the rainy season. Yellow foods, like soybeans and pumpkins, are usually rich in vitamins A and D. Vitamin A can protect the lining in the digestive and respiratory systems, which helps prevent stomach bloating and ulcers. Vitamin D promotes the absorption of calcium and phosphorus, strengthening bones.

White food corresponds with the lung system. White foods

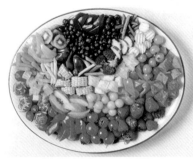

Different colors of foods correspond with different organ systems and seasons.

are best for autumn, providing one of the best remedies for the dryness of the season. Apart from relieving coughing, they also help nourish skin and fight constipation through the promotion of Body Fluids. White foods such as milk, lily bulb, and fish are also recommended by nutritionists as they are rich in protein, yet relatively low in fat.

Black food corresponds with the kidney system. Black foods are best for winter, a season when, according to TCM, one should store energy. The kidney system plays a role in this, and black foods promote and strengthen the kidney system. People with a poor kidney system will miss many of the benefits of the reinforcing foods eaten in winter. Research shows that most black foods are rich in inorganic salt and melanin. Inorganic salt can help promote fluid metabolism and dispel toxins, while melanin restricts nitrosamine, helping to prevent cancer.

2. Food Tastes

The Five Elements theory also states that each of the tastes has certain effects on the body as described below.

Chinese phrase "*wang mei zhi ke* 望梅止渴" (literally, quench one's thirst by thinking of plums) denotes a legendary period during the Eastern Han dynasty (25–220). General Cao Cao (155–220) met the enemy in the course of marching and fought desperately to defeat the enemy, but he failed to find water along the way. While the soldiers were tired and thirsty, their marching speed was very slow. Cao Cao told his soldiers that there was a large plum forest ahead. When the soldiers heard that there were plums, they began to salivate, then as they sped up, their morale was greatly boosted. Of course, they did not get to eat plums, but they were able to find water at last. Hearing and thinking of sour flavored fruit temporarily suppressed the degree of thirst.

Sour. The therapeutic use of sour helps with digestive absorption, resisting fatty foods, and preventing indigestion. It generates fluids and Yin and stops discharge, perspiration, chronic cough, and diarrhea. It also has an astringent effect on emissions, including sperm and frequent urine. It helps the body consolidate essential substances, preventing them from escape. Sour foods can also bring disordered Qi back to normal. Modern research shows sour flavors to be generally cleansing and detoxifying. However, those suffering from ulcer or stones must limit their intake.

Bitter. The phrase "*liang yao ku kou* 良药苦口 " literally means a good medicine tastes bitter. From the historical records, during the development of traditional Chinese herbal medicine, plants with bitter tastes and cold temperatures proved very effective medicines. However, if one applies bitter and cold herbs/plants without a herbalist's instructions, it might lead to some side effects and consequences to the human bodies. Therefore, it is always important to consult professionals to avoid overdosage.

The bitter taste clears away heat and calms, hardens, and dries Dampness. It can control abnormally ascending Qi and purge any pathogenic Heat. In certain combinations, it can also improve the body's Yin. Bitter foods can be used to treat most cases of excess and acute Damp-Heat or Heat-Fire. These foods should be limited if a weakness of Qi and Blood is present.

Sweet. Served to nourish, moisten, moderate and invigorate the body, sweet foods can also regulate Qi, Blood and the function of the viscera. They strengthen deficiency syndromes and alleviate Dryness. Sweet foods work in coordination with the spleen and stomach. They can help relieve pain and spasms and reduce coughs, ulcers, and constipation. An excess of sweets should be avoided when suffering from Damp, Phlegm, and water retention conditions.

Spicy (pungent). This taste disperses and promotes movement of Qi and blood circulation. It stimulates digestion and helps break through blockages. It treats syndromes of the exterior, and expels stagnation of Qi, Blood, and pathogens. Spicy foods must be used carefully as many people cannot tolerate them.

Salty. These foods can promote moisture and have a softening effect. In particular, these foods regulate the moisture balance flow downwards in the body. They also move Qi downward, increase urine and bowel movements, and are used to treat constipation and swelling. They promote the action of the kidney system, allowing beneficial foods to be fully absorbed and functional, and improve concentration. Salty foods soften nodes and masses and disperse accumulations in hardening muscles and glands.

Bland. This taste promotes urination and treats edema.

Applying the Five Elements in the Relationships Between Organs

The generation of the five elements can be used to expound the interdependent relations between the five internal organs. For instance, the vital Essence of the kidney (water) nourishes the liver (wood), which is known as water generating wood. The liver (wood) stores blood to nourish the heart (fire), which is termed wood generating fire. The heat of the heart (fire) warms the spleen (earth), which is called fire generating earth. The spleen (earth) transforms and distributes food's essence to replenish the lung (metal), which is referred to as earth generating metal. The lung (metal) dredges the water passages to help the kidney (water), which is taken as metal generating water.

The restriction of the five elements can be used to explain the inter-restriction of the five viscera. For instance, the lung (metal) disperses and descends so as to restrain the exuberance of the liver (wood), which is known as metal restricting wood. The liver (wood) that functions well smooths and regulates the stagnation of the Qi of the spleen (earth), which is called wood restricting earth. The function of the spleen (earth) plays a role in transporting, distributing, and transforming nutrients and promoting water metabolism and may prevent the overflow of the water of the kidney (water), which is referred to as earth restricting water. The ascending of the kidney (water) can prevent the heart (fire) from hyperactivity, which is explained as water restricting fire.

Chapter Four
The System of Organs and Meridians

Chinese medicine holds the view that the body-mind network is an integrated whole. The conception of the meridians and organ systems reflects this view, representing a landscape of functional relationships that enables the total integration of bodily functions, emotions, mental activities, tissue, sense organs, and environmental influences.

This chapter provides a brief introduction to TCM's view of the organs and their interrelationships. This information is necessary to fully understand how the liver, spleen, kidney, lung, and heart systems influence our mind, outer, and inner body.

The Concept of *Zang-Fu* Organs

In TCM, the organs are organized into two categories: *zang* 脏 (meaning "storage," including the five main *zang* organs, the heart, liver, spleen, lung, and kidney, along with the pericardium) and *fu* 腑 (meaning "passage," including the six *fu* organs, the stomach, gallbladder, *sanjiao*, urinary bladder, large intestine, and small intestine). In this chapter, we will focus on the five main *zang* organs and their linkage with *fu* organs, tissue, and sense organs.

The common physical function of *zang* organs is to produce and store the body's Blood, Fluids and Qi. These organs are responsible for ensuring that the body is full of Essence and Qi, vital and ready for action, and to ensure that flow is not stagnant or blocked. Stagnation or depletion of the Qi or Essence in an organ can affect overall health and may lead to more serious disease.

In the six *fu* organs, *sanjiao*, meaning "triple energizer" or "triple heat," is not one particular anatomical organ. It relates to all muscles (including fascia) and tissues, like a pipe carrying bodily fluids, including lymphatic fluids, circulating them to the whole body.

In Chinese medicine, a *fu* organ is a receptor organ, responsible for receiving food and allowing it to pass through. So the job of the *fu* organs is to receive solid and liquid food, extract the good, and expel the bad.

One vital aspect of the *fu* organs is that there is constant movement. When one organ is full, the others need to be empty and waiting. For instance, when the stomach is full, the intestines should be empty, waiting for food and vice versa.

Another significant concept related to the *fu* organs is that their energy moves downward. For example, since the energy of the stomach needs to be moving downward, if this natural pattern is disturbed and the energy begins moving upward, one might experience indigestion or acid reflux.

It is also important that the *zang* and *fu* organs work together to produce enough nutrition to create and maintain a healthy, harmonized body. When they are working in harmony, the food or liquid that enters the body will be separated into nourishment and waste. The nutrition will be absorbed and distributed into the whole body's systems, while the waste will be excreted.

Organ System Function Connected via the Meridians

The holistic approach is based on the five *zang* organs. These are defined much more broadly than in modern medicine, including not only the organ but its entire functional system, linked via meridians. The meridians are communication lines between all parts of the body—pathways that carry Qi, Blood, and Body Fluids. Let's begin with the heart system.

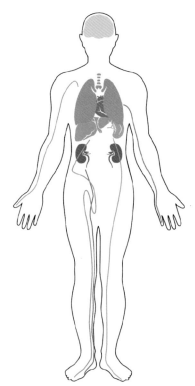

Five organs and five corresponding meridians.

1. The Heart System: Heart, Small Intestine, Blood Vessels, Tongue

TCM believes that heart is the "monarch of the internal organs," the body's "root of life." The heart is in control of the body's physical and psychological functions. It not only governs the blood and circulation (physical heart), but it is also the storehouse of the Spirit (mental heart, some functions of brain). The face is the flower of the heart. The pulse measures the heart's conditions. The tongue is the sprout, and joy is the emotion of the heart. Good blood circulation, a peaceful mind, a glowing complexion, and a hydrated, rosy color on your face are signs of a healthy heart. It is also seen in a pink tongue with free movement, a firm and regular rhythm of the heartbeat, and a comfortable feeling in the chest. Furthermore, the heart determines normal mental activity, a balanced emotional life, clarity of consciousness, a good memory, and sound sleep. For example, when we tense up, we have a red face, quick heartbeat, and sweaty palms. The external and internal relation between heart and small intestine is similar to the correspondence of the Heart Meridian and Small Intestine Meridian, which flow through the Yin side and Yang side of the upper limbs. In modern medicine, it would be roughly equivalent to the circulatory and cranial nervous systems.

Case Study of the Heart System

A 17-year-old female suffered from influenza complicated with myocarditis, with an incomplete right bundle branch block for a period of 5 months. Her main complaint was chest tightness and palpitations. Her pulse was slow with irregular beats, while her tongue was pale with a white coating. At night, she was not able to fall sleep easily, waking up several times during the night, and even having nightmares. During the daytime, she was always tired and could not easily clear her mind.

TCM syndrome diagnosis: Qi and Blood deficiency of the heart and liver, combined with blood stagnation.

Prescription: Eight Treasure Soup (八珍汤) with ginseng, angelica, astragalus, cinnamon twig, and safflower

After a month's treatment, the main symptoms had been mostly reduced. The electrocardiogram examination indicated myocarditis rehabilitation and that the incomplete right bundle branch block had disappeared.

In order to consolidate her treatment for another 2 months, she took functional foods to improve her sleep quality, such as 6 g of longan, 2 g of lingzhi mushroom powder, and 3 g of cooked licorice root. Two months later, the client's physique gradually became normal, allowing her to engage in further studies.

The best foods for her condition: beetroot, cherry, garlic chives

Acupressure points: Neiguan (PC 6), Danzhong (RN 17), Xingjian (LV 2)

---

2. The Liver System: Liver, Gallbladder, Tendons, Eyes

TCM take the liver as "the general" of the whole body. It

regulates a person's feelings of excitement or depression. The liver governs conducting and dispersion and ensures the smooth flow of Qi. This regulates the emotional, digestive, and reproductive function of Qi. The liver is the planning organ in charge of moods, causing emotional ups and downs. The liver stores blood. It is a source of endurance which controls the inherent facilities of the body. The eyes and tears are windows and liquids of the liver. The breasts are the outer territory of the liver. The liver controls the tendons with the outer representation of the nails. The liver emotion can be measured by the degree and frequency of anger. When we have good liver function, Qi will flow freely in the normal speed and direction. Our head and rib regions should be pain free. Our eyes will be shiny, with sharp vision, and our sinews will be flexible. Furthermore, outbursts or feelings of anger will not be a frequent occurrence. Blood is available for use wherever it is needed, and the liver Qi directs the blood to different areas of the body. For example, when we study or require a larger measure of mental energy, the liver directs blood to our head so we can think clearly. When we

Case Study of the Liver System

A 40 year old female who was having a bi-monthly menstruation period found that not only did her menstrual blood turn purple, but also flowed in large volumes. Furthermore, both sides of her lower abdomen were bloated and swollen, and her breasts were sore and painful during each menstrual period. Her face was sallow and pale, her pulse was wiry, and the coating on the sides of her tongue was thin and yellow. All those symptoms were accompanied with mental fatigue and depression.

TCM diagnose: insufficient liver blood, liver Qi stagnant

Prescription: angelica, peony, perilla, tangerine peel, Bupleurum, buddha's hand

After a 5-days treatment, her menstrual symptoms improved. For three consecutive months, there was no similar episode.

The best foods for the condition: wolfberry, prune, shiitake mushrooms

Acupressure points: Sanyinjiao (SP 6), Fengchi (GB 20), Shenmen (HT 7)

participate in sports, the liver sends blood to the limbs and muscles so that our body has adequate blood flow to take action. This blood flow is important for ensuring that the joints and ligaments are well nourished and lubricated. The liver also holds the blood in the organs to prevent bleeding. The external and internal relation between the liver and gallbladder is similar to the correspondence of the Liver Meridian and Gallbladder Meridian, which flow through the Yin side and Yang side of the four limbs. Its functions relate to part of the modern circulatory, peripheral nervous, and digestive systems.

3. The Spleen (Digestive) System: Spleen, Stomach, Muscles, Mouth

"You are what you eat" was a popular saying in the 1990's, although it is only partially true. While "you are what you eat and absorb" would be a better expression of the facts. What you absorb is dependent upon how healthy your spleen system is. The spleen is the source of acquired constitution, meaning all the factors that develop post-natal and are helped more by regulating the digestive system. Directing digestion and absorption, it governs blood flow within the vessels. Therefore we also call the spleen system the "source of Qi and blood." In TCM, the spleen and stomach make up the digestive system, which includes the pancreas, small intestine, and part of the stomach functions as they are known in modern medicine. The spleen is the "Agricultural Bureau" of the body, controlling where energy "seeds" are planted and how the health of the body is harvested. The spleen is the post-natal base of life, meaning once all the congenital factors of the body have been determined, one's health management relies on the spleen to do the rest of the work. When we eat food, our mouth increases saliva by chewing food to help digestion. The lips are the flower of the spleen.

This system controls the muscles and limbs and opens into the pharynx and mouth. Thinking and longing are the emotions of the spleen. The external and internal relationship between spleen and stomach is similar to the correspondence of the Spleen Meridian and Stomach Meridian, which flow through the Yin side and Yang side of the four limbs. It is related to digestion, water metabolism, and the hemopoietin system in modern medicine.

Case Study of the Spleen System

During his inadvertent diet, a 50 year old male suffered from acute bacterial dysentery. His stool contained pus and blood and he was constipated (feeling he needed to pass stool urgently, but could not do so). Because he had been diagnosed with chronic colitis, he received modern medical and Chinese medical treatments. There was still mucus in the stool and he had a feeling of falls and swelling on anus area, conditions that recurred for more than 4 months.

The most current symptoms were frequent episodes of diarrhea, especially after eating greasy food, accompanied with a reddish tongue with a light yellow coating and a slow and slippery pulse.

TCM diagnosis: insufficient spleen, digestive dysfunction

Prescription: ginseng, poria, and ovate atractylodes powder. For children, ginseng, cooked pearl barley, burned hawthorn, lablab (dolichos seed), scutellaria (*qing pi*), ash (*huang qin*), ovate atractylodes, poria

After the 7-day treatment, most of the symptoms were under control. He continued a course of scutellaria, ash, add medicated leaven (*shen qu*), blast-fried ginger (*pao jiang*) for a month to assure his complete recovery.

The best foods for the condition: yam, nutmeg, lotus seed

Acupressure points: Hegu (LI 4), Zusanli (ST 36), Tianshu (ST 25)

4. The Lung System: Lung, Large Intestine, Skin and Body Hair, Nose

TCM describes the lung as the "prime minister of the body," because it works hard to protect the other organs. The lung receives messages from the heart and administers these signals throughout the body, especially producing and regulating the body's Qi. The lung's function of governing respiration is related to the exchange of O_2 (oxygen) and CO_2 (carbon dioxide). The lung is the intermediary organ between the internal body and the external environment. The process of inhaling (Qi down and in) and exhaling (Qi up and out) influences all the Qi movements within our body. It controls the circulation and regulates the body's upper portion metabolism of fluids. The lung controls the skin, and the system opens into the larynx and nose. Worry and sadness are the emotions of the lungs.

The external and internal relation between the lungs and large intestine is similar to the correspondence of the Lung Meridian and Large Intestine Meridian, which flow through the Yin side and Yang side of the four limbs. The approximate modern equivalent is the respiratory system and processes involved in fluid regulation.

Case Study of the Lung System

A 50 year old male with continuous uncontrolled coughing, sometimes even an asthmatic cough or drowning cough. It combined with white mucus, and his throat was itchy. He had white tongue with a thick coat and a slippery pulse.

TCM diagnose: Cold Phlegm obstructing the lung, disturbed lung opening

Prescription: fresh ginger, scallion bulb, cinnamon twig, almond, black bean sauce, mustard seed

After 10 days of treatment, the cough was controlled.

The best foods for the condition: pear, gingko nut, tremella

Acupressure points: Lieque (LU 7), Taixi (KI 3), Taiyuan (LU 9)

5. The Kidney System: Kidney, Urinary Bladder, Bone, Ears and Lower Orifices

The kidney is responsible for the body's overall constitution and is the congenital base of life. It is a storage facility for good essence, and it governs the growth and development of the body and the reproductive systems. The kidneys, an important source of Yin and Yang, can influence all the organ systems and create Yin-Yang balance. They governs water metabolism, which can be seen in two ways. The first reuses Body Fluids and dispels waste. The second promotes water metabolism for other organs, especially the lungs and spleen, to maintain excellent nourishment without swelling. The kidneys' governing of the reception and transformation of Qi helps facilitate deeper breathing and allows the body to store some extra Qi. The kidney system controls the bones, producing marrow, and opens into the ears and two lower orifices. If a person has sufficient kidney Yin and Yang Qi, they will have sensitive hearing and firm, strong teeth. Hair is the flower of the kidneys. Gorgeous, rich, shining long hair can be a reflection of strong kidney essence. Fear and fright are the emotions of the kidney. The external and internal relationship between kidney and urinary bladder is similar to the correspondence of the Kidney Meridian and Urinary Bladder Meridian, which flow through the Yin side and Yang side of the four limbs. It can be seen as equivalent to the urogenital and endocrine system, as well as part of the nervous system.

Case Study of the Kidney System

A female, 34 years old, suffered from frequent urinary problems, day and night for more than a month. The number of recurrences was difficult to recall. The urine color was slightly yellow, with no feeling of heat or burning when passing water. It was accompanied by a backache and sore legs, along with a heavy vaginal discharge. Her pulse was deep and thin, and her tongue pale with a thin white coat.

TCM diagnose: kidney Qi weakness, less hold function

Prescription: astragalus, bugbane rhizome (cimicifugae), euryale (*qian shi*), raspberry, alpinia, walnut juglans regia L., cinnamon bark

After 12 days of this herbal decoction, she improved greatly.

The best foods for the condition: walnut, schisandra berry, sword bean

Acupressure points: Shenshu (BL 23), Guanyuan (RN 4), Baihui (DU 20)

Paired *Zang-Fu* Organs

From the analysis above, we know that one *zang* organ will pair with one *fu* organ. The pairing systems of *zang* and *fu* organs developed as a result of three observations.

Proximity. For instance, the liver is close to the gallbladder, the stomach is close to the spleen, and the kidney is close to the urinary bladder.

Patterns. These were observed over thousands of years. For instance, it was noted that the lung and large intestine share a special relationship. When one showed patterns of disharmony, the other was often affected, so by treating one, you could affect the other.

Meridians. These organ pairs are linked by meridians. It is also important that the *zang* and *fu* organs work together to produce enough nutrition to create and maintain a healthy, harmonized body. For instance the Lung Meridian begins inside the middle belly area and runs down to connect with the large intestine. The Lung Meridian then passes through the diaphragm, all the way to the lung. The surface of the Lung and Large Intestine Meridian line also branch together, traveling on corresponding sides of the upper limbs. Hence the lung and large intestine are intimately connected through the meridians.

Main Paired Organs in TCM	
Zang Organ	*Fu* Organ
Heart	Small intestine
Liver	Gallbladder
Spleen	Stomach
Lung	Large intestine
Kidney	Urinary bladder

The *zang* and *fu* organs are classified into pairs.

Self-Assessing Your Five Organ Systems
In order to understand more about your organ systems, you can do a self-assessment below. The following questionnaire will help you discover which organ system you should be most concerned about.

1. Questions Relating to the Heart System
Do you have trouble sleeping at night?
☐ yes   ☐ no

Do you have heart palpitations?
☐ yes   ☐ no

Do you have sweaty hands?
☐ yes   ☐ no

Are you forgetful?
☐ yes   ☐ no

Do you have circulatory problems?
☐ yes   ☐ no

Do you feel nervous often?
☐ yes   ☐ no

Do you frequently get ulcers on your tongue?
☐ yes   ☐ no

Is your sleep often disturbed by nightmares or stressful dreams?
☐ yes   ☐ no

Do you have an irregular heartbeat?
☐ yes   ☐ no

Do you often feel unhappy?
☐ yes   ☐ no

2. Questions Relating to the Liver System

Do you regularly experience premenstrual syndrome (PMS) symptoms?
☐ yes   ☐ no

Are your nails brittle or cracked?
☐ yes   ☐ no

Do you often feel moody & cranky?
☐ yes   ☐ no

Do you have a high stress lifestyle?
☐ yes   ☐ no

Do your eyes tear frequently?
☐ yes   ☐ no

Do you often feel irritable or restless?
☐ yes   ☐ no

Do you regularly experience blurred vision and dry, red, and/or swollen eyes?

□ yes   □ no

Do you have tendon problems?

□ yes   □ no

Do you often get migraine headaches?

□ yes   □ no

Do you often feel uncomfortable in your rib area (on both sides) and/or top of your head and temple regions?

□ yes   □ no

3. Questions Relating to the Spleen System

Do you have severe food allergies or do you get food poisoning more than twice a year?

□ yes   □ no

Do you have sensitivities to certain foods?

□ yes   □ no

Do you often feel bloated after eating?

□ yes   □ no

Do you have heartburn?

□ yes   □ no

Do you often have diarrhea?

□ yes   □ no

Do you frequently have bad breath?

□ yes   □ no

Do you often have an upset stomach or nausea?

□ yes   □ no

Do you bruise easily?

□ yes   □ no

Do you dislike the wet season or damp weather?
☐ yes   ☐ no

Do you have muscle problems (weakness, tightness, stiffness, knots, easy muscle tearing)?
☐ yes   ☐ no

4. Questions Relating to the Lung System

Are you particularly susceptible to colds or flu?
☐ yes   ☐ no

Do you frequently have a cough or asthma?
☐ yes   ☐ no

Do you often experience shortness of breath?
☐ yes   ☐ no

Do you have nasosinusitis?
☐ yes   ☐ no

Do you feel sad often?
☐ yes   ☐ no

Do you often have a sore or tickling throat, mucus, or regularly need to clear your throat?
☐ yes   ☐ no

Do you have hay fever?
☐ yes   ☐ no

Do you often have skin issues?
☐ yes   ☐ no

Do you smoke?
☐ yes   ☐ no

Do you have constipation?
☐ yes   ☐ no

5. Questions Relating to the Kidney System

Do your ears ring?

☐ yes   ☐ no

Do you experience pain in your back, knees or heels?

☐ yes   ☐ no

Do you have infertility or a low sperm count?

☐ yes   ☐ no

Do you have a low sexual drive?

☐ yes   ☐ no

Do you suffer from frequent urges to urinate?

☐ yes   ☐ no

Do you suffer from hair loss?

☐ yes   ☐ no

Do your bones or teeth break easily?

☐ yes   ☐ no

Do you experience menopausal symptoms?

☐ yes   ☐ no

Do you find it difficult to completely empty your bladder?

☐ yes   ☐ no

Do you have fear or panic attacks?

☐ yes   ☐ no

The category that has attracted the most "yes" answers is the organ system you should give attention to first. After you have strengthened or regulated your weak organ system for at least two months, take the quiz again. If you are lucky enough to have not answered "yes" more than 3 times in any one category, congratulations! Your diet and lifestyle are relatively healthy!

The Chinese View of Organs as a Whole System

We first need to explore some fundamental differences between TCM's view of the form and function of organs and the modern anatomical or medical description. For instance, when referring to the liver, in modern medicine, it points to the anatomical organ itself and its function. In Chinese medicine, when we refer to the liver, this includes the whole organ system: the structure and function of the organ, the paired organ, related meridians, the tissue, related sense organs, emotions unique to that organ, sound associated with the organ, and exterior appearance related to the organ.

Therefore, if the liver system becomes imbalanced, issues might manifest as a problem in any of the areas mentioned above. A good TCM practitioner will recognize the symptoms and prevent a more serious disease from occurring.

The Chinese View of Meridians as an Overall Network

Each organ has its own pathway system to carry and transport materials to every cell and extremity of the body. The pathways consist of meridians or channels, which branch out into collaterals. It is on the superficial meridian where we find the acupuncture points. The deep collaterals have points that can be influenced by breath control and Qigong exercises or other manual modalities. The meridians are where we apply Tuina (massage), acupressure or acupuncture, cupping, and Gua Sha to rebalance the body.

The meridians have a close relationship with the organ systems. They are the passages by which the *zang*, or major organs (for example, the heart), and *fu*, or secondary organs (for example, the small intestine), connect with one another.

The relationships between the liver, heart, spleen, lung, and

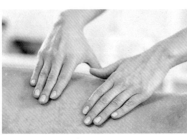

kidney show these connections. In the meridian system, the Liver Meridian and the Gallbladder Meridian run through the heart. The Liver Meridian runs on both sides of the stomach, which is part of the spleen system. The Kidney Meridian ascends and runs through the liver, the

Tuina massage.

Liver Meridian ascends to the lung, and so on. By means of these interconnecting meridians, the five systems maintain relative balance and coordination.

However you can impact the collaterals and the related organ by stimulating acupoints or skin zones on the meridians. The meridians will also have branches that are less closely linked to other organs. The organs are connected with surface points on the body along these lines of energy. Therefore the entire body, inside and out, comprises one of the overall human body systems, which moves energy and regulates health.

Chapter Five
The Material Foundation of the Body

Qi (vital energy), Essence, Blood, and Body Fluids are the basic materials that form the foundation of the body and sustain human life. In this chapter, we look at each material to gain a better understanding of the relationship between Qi, Essence, Blood, and Body Fluids.

Concept & Formation of Qi

Qi is a fundamental concept in traditional Chinese culture, and it is a part of everything that exists. It is everywhere in all the wonders of the universe. Everything you can see, feel, and experience contains Qi. It is the energy, vitality, or life-process that flows in and around all of us.

The concept of Qi is at the roots of TCM theory. Qi is the most fundamental material constituting the human body and the foundation for the functioning of the body's organs and meridians.

Qi is universal and invisible, and it has great power. It flows through the whole body because of its strength. The body has two sources of Qi. One is the innate vital substance we inherit from our parents before birth. The other is acquired from our environment, including the air, water, and food in the natural world.

Essence is another essential material of the body, stored in the kidneys. Kidney Essence is inherited from our family, similar to DNA, and it heavily influences development. After birth, Essence is accumulated through nutrients. It comes from the mother's breast milk, and later from healthy food and oxygen. Qi, Blood, and Body Fluids form part of the Essence to be stored in the body for further development.

Qi and Essence can be exchanged. Stored Essence can be converted into Qi for daily activity. If you are highly active, Essence is used as Qi. If you are calm and relaxed, Qi can be stored as Essence for future use.

Qi is created from oxygen inhaled during the breathing process, food essence, and the original Qi you are born with.

The lungs play a very important role in this process, because your breathing processes enrich your Qi. Without good breathing habits, the quality and quantity of Qi can be affected. The idea of food essence comes from the TCM concept of the spleen, which refers to the group of organs with digestive functions, including the spleen, pancreas, and part of the small intestine. The spleen transforms and transports your nutrients into "clear Qi." You are born with an original Qi (kidney Essence's Qi form), which is stored in your kidneys. We can, however, have significant influence on the digestive system as we have personal choices regarding what we consume. Therefore, according to the Five Elements Theory, if you take care of your digestive system, your lung Qi can be strong. Not only that, but your whole body Qi and Essence can be stronger too.

Classification of Qi

There are four types of Qi:

Original Qi (*yuan qi*) is inherited and enriched by foods. However, Chest Qi, Defensive Qi, and Nutrient Qi all depend on the ecosystem and diet. As such, if we have a deficiency of Qi somewhere in the body, TCM will always start by addressing the diet.

Chest Qi (*zong qi*) originates mainly from the oxygen inhaled during exercise and from food essence. It is predominately stored in the Danzhong point between the lungs and heart. Chest Qi keeps the airways open for the lungs. If it can effectively flow to the throat, singing and talking for long periods of time without discomfort will be easy. For the heart, Chest Qi helps to warm the heart and promotes efficient blood circulation.

Defensive Qi (*wei qi*) comes from Yang food that is Warm, Hot,

Spicy, or Sweet. If energy is not moving, add some spice to bring energy to the head. If you are weak, eat something Warm and Sweet to bring up energy levels. Defensive Qi can also make your temperature stable. It allows your body to sweat if it is hot or to close pores if it is cold, therefore keeping your temperature stable. If there is an epidemic or flu spreading, defensive Qi will fight to stop you from getting sick (In western medicine, this aligns with the notion of the immune system).

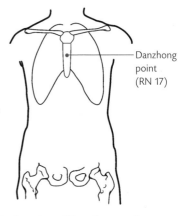

The location of Danzhong point.

Nutrient Qi (*ying qi*) originates from nutrition of food transformed by the spleen and stomach. It is the component part within the blood flowing throughout the body. Nutrient Qi circulates in the blood vessels and is transformed into blood to nourish the whole body.

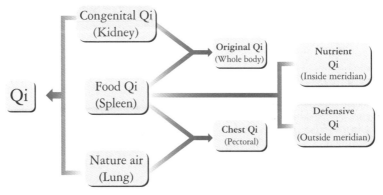

Production, movements and function of various types of Qi.

Movement Style of Qi—Up, Down, In, Out
The various functions of Qi are all performed by its movement. The basic movements of Qi are in four forms: ascending, descending, inwards, and outwards. These movements of Qi are vital to life and keep the body functioning effectively.

The actions of inhaling and exhaling are an example of Qi moving. Exhalation is the exit and ascent of Qi, while inhalation is the descending and entering movement of Qi. For the lung to function, we must move Qi up and out by exhaling and move Qi in and down by practicing deep inhaling. This is seen in Qigong, martial arts, meditation, and yoga, which are all combined with breathing techniques to make them more powerful and effective.

The five major organs (five organ systems) all harmonize using the four movements of Qi. They are divided into three levels, and pairs of organs work together from different levels in the body. As Qi increases in one, it decreases in the other. Three levels of *sanjiao* (triple energizer) are: upper energizer heart and lung, middle energizer spleen and stomach, and lower energizer liver and kidney.

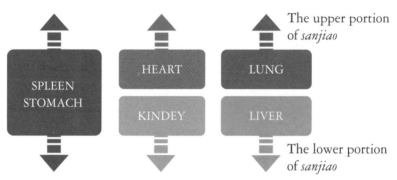

Three levels of *sanjiao*.

We can see how the pairs of organs work together to harmonize the body, also noting the five organs aligned with the five elements, wood, water, metal, fire and earth.

1. Heart (Fire) and Kidney (Water)—Water Can Harmonize Fire

If your heart rate increases, and you have a flushed face or heart palpitations, it can be calmed and cooled with water. Drink room temperature water and lie down, thinking about being by a water source such as the ocean or lake.

2. Lung (Metal) and Liver (Wood)—Metal Can Control and Shape Wood

If you become anxious or irritated, breathe deeply to help reduce the feeling of anxiety. Our normal breathing rate should be from 16-18 times per minute, but if we are anxious it can be up to 30 times per minute. It is essential to bring the breathing rate down and to feel calm. Lie down and breathe deeply and slowly to lower the speed.

3. Spleen (Earth) and Stomach (Earth)—the Digestive System Is Earth, the Mother of All Elements

Earth does not need to harmonize with the other elements, but with the sky and universe. The spleen and stomach are in the same level and influence the entire organ system. Though in the middle, the spleen sends energy up, while the stomach sends energy down. Eating well and having a good, stable digestive system can therefore harmonize the whole body. The functions of breathing and digestion can be used to manage many things in life, including our metabolism, hormones, and emotions.

Blood and Body Fluids

Blood and Body Fluids are also fundamental materials of the body. However, they are more visible and material than Qi. Blood and Body Fluids belong to Yin, while Qi belongs to Yang.

Blood is one of the essential substances that makes up the human body and maintains its life activities. It is a red fluid that flows in the vessels, rich in nutrition. The spleen, lung, heart, and kidney organ systems are vital for the production of Blood.

Body Fluids are called *jin ye* in Chinese. This word is composed of two characters, the first meaning "moist" or "saliva," which indicates anything that is liquid, and the second meaning "fluid," indicating fluids contained in living organisms (i.e., those found in vegetables and fruit). The stomach, spleen, small intestine, and large intestine are necessary for the production of Body Fluids.

Both Blood and Body Fluids are liquid. Blood is rich in nutrients and red in color, whereas Body Fluids are transparent and have both thin and thick density. In TCM, the formation of blood is a combination of Nutrient Qi and Body Fluids.

Nutrient Qi is formed from our daily consumption of food and drink, and also dependent on the temperature and taste of food. Water, soup, fruit, and herbal tea make up Body Fluids. If these are sufficient, the digestive system can function properly and ensure that the lung and heart can put blood and oxygen into the system. The lung and heart functions help us to make essential blood.

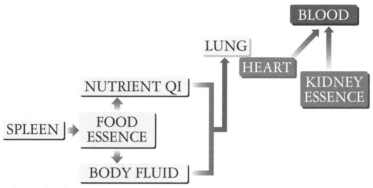

Relationship between organs and fundamental materials of the body.

Essence also makes Blood. The kidneys store Essence, which produces marrow in our bones, brain, and spine. Marrow in the spine can make Blood, which is then stored in the liver and then circulated around the body for use. The kidney stores Essence, and the liver stores Blood. As they share the same source, Essence and Blood can transform into each other.

The "home for the Blood" is known as the "meridian vessels." All meridian vessels are linked together in a network that endlessly circulates blood around the body. The specific structures for efficient circulation are the structures of the fourteen meridians connecting the internal organs.

The fourteen meridian structure consists of twelve meridians, plus the Yang meridian of *du* and Yin meridian of *ren*. The heart and lungs also promote blood circulation using their energy, with the heart Qi pushing blood out and the lung Qi bringing blood in. The liver also plays a role, as the liver is the mother of the heart and is the secondary organ to promote circulation. The liver and spleen's function is to hold the blood to prevent the body from losing blood, slowing down, or bruising, so that blood can circulate effectively.

In Western medicine, the most important role of blood is for circulation. In TCM, the Blood has one function, to nourish and moisturize the entire body system, since organs, tissues, and nerves all need sufficient blood to function. At the same time, TCM believes that Blood is very important to the emotions and spirit. For example, if a woman has emotional problems, we will address the Blood first to ensure a more effective treatment. If a patient is diagnosed with Alzheimer's, we will first increase blood circulation to the brain through food and herbs.

The "home for metabolism of Body Fluids" is the triple energizer. Body Fluids are moved by the energy of the lungs, spleen, and kidneys. The triple energizer therefore acts like a pipe, and the Body Fluids are circulated inside via the process of formation, transportation, and excretion.

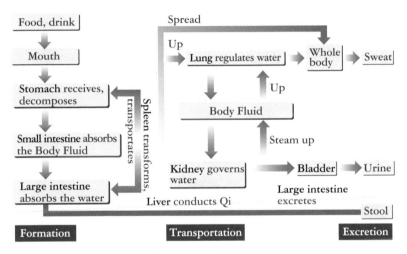

Formation, transportation and excretion of Body Fluid.

There are two types of Body Fluids, one being basic liquid, and the other being nutrient liquid. Basic liquid depends on how much we sweat or talk (saliva), with the body adjusting how much liquid is required accordingly. For example, in summer, if we are active or have a job that requires lots of talking, we will need to drink 6 to 8 cups of water per day to replenish the Body Fluids. In winter, we sweat less, so may reduce the quantity of liquid we need to drink. Nutrient liquid depends on how we feel and what our sense organs indicate, such as being thirsty, or having dry skin and scalp. For example, people who are dry may find that their hands and feet will become dry, rough and crack easily in the winter or autumn. If they experience this, they need to increase nutrient liquid intake, which can be done by making soup from roots or fresh beans and increasing the intake of seeds and nuts in the diet. Another way to judge if you have enough Body Fluids is to check urine and stool. Dark brown or dark yellow urine indicate more Body Fluids are needed and liquid intake should be increased. If someone is constipated or has diarrhea, Body Fluids will need to be adjusted accordingly.

We remove waste from our bodies to detox in different ways. One way is through lung waste, created by talking and sweating. When we talk, waste is removed from the body so it can be used as a detoxing method. We also sweat to remove waste, which we can increase through breathing exercises and physical activities. The spleen and kidney also remove waste carried by Body Fluids, as they are responsible for urination and bowel movements. Urination is the most important excretion by which waste leaves the body. If you do not urinate, it can be highly problematic for the body.

The Relationship between Qi, Blood, and Body Fluids

The illustration shows the Qi army general leading the Blood and Body Fluids. Blood and Body Fluids are the mother protecting the Qi.

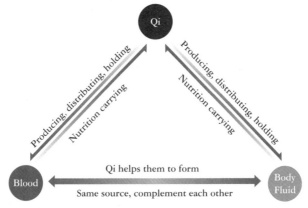

Relationship between Qi, Blood and Body Fluid.

For someone who has anemia, TCM prescribes iron-rich food to strengthen the Blood and energy-dense food to strengthen Qi so that both Blood and Qi are addressed. This would especially be the case for a quiet person who needs to strengthen Qi. The increased energy can help the absorption of iron-rich and blood-strengthening food. Toning Blood and toning Qi work together to achieve the best results.

A dry person who can never quench their thirst or increase

moisture also needs to think of Qi, Body Fluids and Blood. We cannot only focus on increasing fluid intake, as this may make no difference or lead to water retention. If increasing liquid does not help, it indicates that the Qi relationship with Body Fluids is not in balance. TCM advises both toning Qi and adding more liquid, so that Qi can help the liquid go to the appropriate area of the body. External treatment can also be used, such as massage or tapping. For example, if someone is suffering from swelling in the ankle, they can use massage and warmth therapy to open the energy so the Qi can move. As such, water and fluid will follow, moving excess water back into circulation.

Qi, Blood, and Body Fluids complement each other and have multifaceted relationships with the internal organ systems. Qi has the function of promoting Blood and Body Fluid circulation and metabolism, warming and protecting the body, and holding the body's liquid materials and internal organs in place. It also is responsible for aiding the transformation of nutrition, Essence, Blood, and Body Fluids from one to another. The kidney, spleen, and lung are important for the production of Qi. Dr. Fei Boxiong, a classically trained scholar and famous physician from the Qing dynasty, noted the importance of these interrelationships, saying, "The five *zang* and six *fu* organs produce Qi and Blood. When Qi and Blood are full of vigor, they nourish the *zang-fu* organs."

Blood and Body Fluids are inseparable from Qi, and Qi infuses life into Blood and Body Fluids. However, Blood and Body Fluids are much denser and unlike Qi, which cannot change into an invisible form.

Clinically, Blood and Body Fluids help each other. For instance, if you have swelling during hot summer or from a long distance flight, blood circulation can be regulated to help move the Body Fluids and reduce swelling. To do so, increase the quantity of food such as black fungus (wood ear mushroom), gingko nuts, saffron, or safflower, which are Neutral and Blood strengthening, promoting blood circulation. Or use red ginseng under the tongue or in tea to speed up circulation for the heart and brain. You can also do some outdoor exercise to increase Qi.

Effective blood circulation and strengthening Qi are also key to speeding up metabolism.

The Relationship between Essence, Qi, and Spirit

There are three parts of life, Qi, Essence, and Spirit. If we know how to store energy, accumulate Essence, and harmonize emotions/mental state/Spirit, then we can achieve holistic health. If we can balance all three, each life stage will be more harmonized and stable. To do so, we need to address two levels.

Psychological condition. Our invisible Qi needs to be harmonized with our visible Essence (brain and spine) so it can pass through generation to generation via the reproductive system. Also visible part of life activities directly impact mental state, such as daily activities, responses, emotions, and so forth.

Physical condition. This denotes the Qi and Essence and how they can support the psychological part of the body. If Qi and Essence can strengthen each other, then we can stay balanced and achieve optimal health.

Chapter Six
Knowing Our Constitution

What is the first thing you do when you wake up in the morning? Drink a cup of coffee? Drink a cup of warm water? Open the bedroom window? Plan your new day? Decide what to eat for breakfast? Half awake, still tired, you run out of the door ...

In Chinese, we say "An hour in the morning is worth two in the evening." No matter whether it is a healthy lifestyle, a blueprint for a career development, or finding some new scientific knowledge, planning before the day starts is always important.

Here, let's focus on our health. For me, the first thing one should do is drinking a cup of warm water. Then you should not only open the window of the soul, but also opens the window of the house for refreshment. How do we open the window of the heart? You can stretch your neck and chest 3 times. Or you can extend your arms and clap your hands for 20 seconds, walking forward like a soldier, assuring your arms and legs are raised high for 20 steps. If you still have a minute of spare time, you can massage the top of your head for 20 seconds. All these activities can wake your mind and body by increasing Yang energy as you adapt to the sun rising.

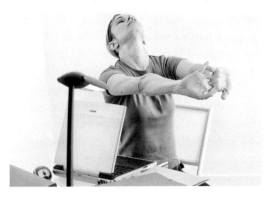

Stretch your body once
every two hours at work.

I plan my breakfast one night in advance. I choose a variety of breakfast foods each day, then after 3 or 4 days, I repeat the cycle. I will provide a two-day menu as a demonstration (see details on pages 169-172 in Part Three).

At work, we must adjust the distance between our body and the computer or operating platform according to ergonomic principles. This arrangement has long been the way to protect the spine, especially the cervical spine. Don't bend over, and don't remain in a sitting position for too long. Stand up and move, drink some water, and stretch your body once every two hours.

Lunch should contain a variety of foods, assuring a combination of meat and vegetables, soup, soft and solid foods, and so forth. After lunch, some people choose to relax and take a break, while others go for a short walk. Compared with the other two meals, dinner can be simpler, such as two dishes and one soup. It is best to have dinner between 6 pm and 7 pm, and not to end dinner too late.

There is a Chinese saying, "Stroll for a hundred steps after a meal, and you would be able to live up to 99." It is best to have half an hour stroll after a meal, swinging the arms and massaging the abdomen 300 times.

If you plan to fall asleep at 11 pm, try to drink less water after 9 pm. If you want to drink some liquids after dinner and between bedtime, this should be regulated according to the season and your sleep patterns. For example, in spring time and during summer, you can drink mung bean and pearl barley soup, chrysanthemum tea, chamomile tea, or other similar drinks. You can chose to drink some flower tea in autumn and winter, such as osmanthus tea, rose tea, tangerine peel tea, or citron tea.

Body constitution comprises our physical state, including the morphology, function of our internal systems, and metabolism, along with our mental and spiritual states. As we pass through life, everyone's physical constitution goes through periods of relative balance and imbalance, for example, passing from Hot to Cold or Dry to Damp. Imbalance of our physical constitution can mark a transitional stage, when we are shifting away from health towards disorder, but before disease develops. Therefore, maintaining balance in our physical constitution can prevent or lessen disease and promote recovery from illness.

Traditional Chinese medicine strives to balance the physical constitution, mitigate shock from the outside environment, and dissolve toxic substances within the body.

Where Does Your Constitution Come from

Before we talk about using TCM methods for classifying different constitutions, we first need to better understand the concept. What exactly is constitution? Where does it come from? How can it be influenced?

The features of one's constitution can be detected in three areas: the physical build of the person, the body's internal functions, and the psychological state. It also depends on the stage of life the person is facing, such as puberty or menopause.

The constitution has two origins: congenital natural disposition and post-natal lifestyle (i.e., nature and nurture).

Many factors influence the formation of the constitution, such as the parents' health, physically and mentally, the time of conception, and the mother's condition during pregnancy. These are all part of the congenital natural disposition of one's constitution.

However, most of the influence comes from our own actions and lifestyle. We can examine these influences in six categories: diet, life balance, environment, marriage and conception, illness, and age and gender.

1. Diet

There are actually three contributing categories in this key area. The first is basic healthy food that helps the body maintain itself on a daily basis. The second is food for pleasure. The last is food for the purpose of healing, reducing risks of illness, and maintaining and promoting high quality of life.

Modern nutritional science is researching this last category now more than ever, as our bodies fight to stay in good health in a fast-paced and changing world. However, "functional food" or food as medicine, as we call this last category, has had 5,000 years of history in TCM.

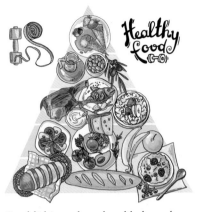

Establishing a broad and balanced diet.

The aim of a healthy diet is to establish a broad and balanced base, making foods digestible and suit the individual. If we always drink or eat gluttonously, for instance drinking beer/soft drinks or taking bigger meals, it will enlarge the stomach.

Establishing unhealthy eating habits, such as emotional eating, picky and rapid eating, skipping breakfast, having late and heavy dinners, eating while walking or watching TV, or eating junk foods, desserts, and snacks, can disturb the digestive motion, decrease the digestive enzyme secretion, and lower the natural ability to digest and absorb.

It is advisable to eat three meals at a relatively regular time of day, and eating until approximately 70% to 80% full, especially for dinner. As the saying goes, eat breakfast like a king, lunch like a commoner, and dinner like a beggar. While taking a meal, allot 20 minutes to half an hour, focusing only on the food. To get the digestive system fully prepared before eating, take care to chew the foods thoroughly. It's important to chew 20 times, then swallow slowly, which assures that saliva will be mixed well with the foods, saving the stomach effort when it receives the foods. The chewing process also influences our Gallbladder Meridians and prepares sufficient bile.

It will be economical and time saving to build up healthy food habits at a younger age, so that in our middle and later ages, we will suffer from less discomfort. When we become parents, we should teach our children healthy food habits before they turn six.

As we know, there are two constitutions, called Cold and Hot.

When we are young or middle aged, the Cold or Hot constitution may only display slight symptoms in the winter or summer, but in other seasons, we display a Neutral constitution. As we age, or if we had severe diseases that we recover from, it will be combined with a decreased power of energy. It displays weakness and Cold or weakness and Heat at same time. "Weakness and Cold" is a state alternatively known as "energy and Yang weakness with cold feelings," while "weakness and Heat" is a state that is also called "Body Fluid and Blood shortage with Heat feelings." Therefore at this stage, you should chose food that can tone Qi and Yang to add warmness, or food that can tone Yin and Blood to add coolness. By combining those two kinds of food therapies, you will gradually achieve better results.

According to World Health Organization surveys, Japan is one of the countries with the lowest obesity rate in the world, and lowest of all developed countries. It's even more amazing that the Japanese people don't participate in sports activities often, but they live longer. Behind these anomalies is the secret of their eating habits. Whether it's eating raw, steamed, or stewed food or applying light cooking, or eating more fish to receive nutritional benefits, or eating less food, or eating food slower, it's all a part of healthy eating. Eating fish should also be divided into seasons. Eat elasmobranch fish in spring, salmon in summer, saury in the fall, and bluefin tuna in winter.

2. Life Balance

Constitution is influenced by how one balances periods of work, stress, and activity with those of calmness, quiet, and reflection. If we work long hours and do not have enough time to relax, or sometimes not even to eat or sleep properly, our constitution will be out of balance. In TCM, there's a law of the right time for everything, and timing and schedule are crucial to maintaining a healthy constitution.

For instance, the time for the paired *zang-fu* organs of the gallbladder and liver is between 11 pm and 3 am. During this period, the gallbladder and liver are re-harmonizing and detoxifying themselves. This process is crucial to a restful sleep. It is also the best time to readjust the metabolism, since the liver stimulates the detoxification process of the other organs. Drinking alcohol and

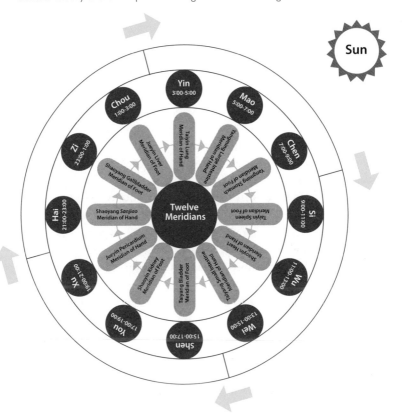

Relationship between the twelve periods of day and meridians.

sleeping very late will multiply the harm to your liver. Since our gallbladder is most active between 11 pm to 1 am, it is crucial to fall asleep at this time. The Huang Emperor initiated time designated by the Heavenly Stems and Earthly Branches, while the midnight and noon were named as *zi* and *wu* time, which are the turning points from Yin to Yang, Yang to Yin. If we can stabilize our moods and have peace of mind, it will charge the energy up, and half the work will produce double the results.

The stomach's peak time is between 7 am and 9 am, so your digestive Fire (as defined in TCM) is strongest at this time. Since an assimilation of nutrients is most effective between these hours, it is essential to eat a nourishing breakfast during these hours, in order to boost your energy for the day.

3. Environment

Our surroundings affect our constitution, whether those influences are physical (such as weather, pollution, or seasonal changes) or social/emotional (friends, co-workers, and support systems).

Influences from the natural environmental are not only external to us, since they affect the water and food we put into our bodies. Therefore a healthy environment can protect your constitution.

4. Marriage and Conception

After marriage, partners can affect each others' constitutions. A balance of sexual activity is needed to maintain harmony in a marriage. Too little or too much can influence the balance of the body.

Similarly, when women do not conceive, they also show signs of disharmony in the body, because pregnancy is a natural cycle in a woman's lifetime. The absence of pregnancy can cause the under-development of some meridian systems. Even women who decide not to breastfeed can show signs of blockage in the Liver and Stomach Meridians due to the inability to access certain meridians connected to the process of releasing milk from the body. Frequent pregnancy is also a disharmonizing situation for women with weaker constitutions.

5. Illness

Disease and other harmful conditions can change one's constitution. During the period when people fall ill, their body Qi, Blood, and the Yin and Yang of their viscera are disturbed because of the harmful pathogenic factors. Normally, when one recovers, these changes also mend gradually and should not alter the overall constitution.

However, certain special circumstances, such as a serious and

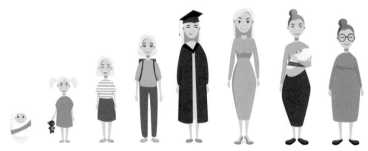

Constitution is subject to changes during different periods of life.

long-term illness, can cause lasting damage. If the body is not sufficiently restored and balanced after illness, the body constitution becomes weak. For example, if a patient experiences long-term chronic hemorrhages or overly heavy menstruation, it can easily cause excessive uterine Qi deficiency, forming a weak constitution.

A metaphor for the relationship between the cause and type of an illness and the physical constitution is that the pathological reaction process is like an oil painting. The constitution is the background color on the drawing board. The pathological changes triggered by the specific cause of the illness are the details of the oil painting, and the type of illness is the overall impression or effect of the oil painting.

6. Age and Gender

The constitution of infants features puerile Yin-Yang and tender organ systems, especially the digestive and respiratory systems. If an infant has a weak constitution, diligent care can gradually bring about a shift to a healthy, vigorous constitution in adolescence. By contrast, even if the original constitution is good, poor nutrition and habits in childhood can cause the constitution to become increasingly weak in adolescence.

Similarly, constitution is subject to changes during other periods of life. During one's retirement years, kidney Essence is decreased and Yin-Yang balance levels are downcast, resulting in a tendency toward fear, fatigue, and lonely feelings, which shows a weakening of the constitution. The body functions, as well as the structure of each system, progressively recede during this phase.

Menopause marks a period of transition from adulthood into old age. It involves both women and men, but in women it is more obvious. It has a different effect on each individual, based on the degree of balance in the constitution.

The properties of Yin and Yang are different. Similarly, the properties of the male and female body are different. Males build up more Yang, showing tall, strong, and stable physical characteristics. Their constitutions are more Hot and strong. Females build up more Yin, so that their outward appearance is slender, soft, and supple. Their constitutions are more Cold and weak. Therefore, men and women have many differences in their physiological functions, and their psychological state and coping abilities are different too. This is determined by gender.

Self-Assessing Your Body Constitution

Here, I provide tools for assessing your body constitution. As noted
earlier, the constitution is a major concept in TCM, and it must
be taken into consideration when selecting foods. Two women in
the same age group can have completely different food therapies,
because their constitutions are opposite. If Woman A has a Hot
constitution, she needs Cool or Cold foods to balance her body,
while Woman B, with a Cold constitution, needs to harmonize with
Warm or Hot foods.

The following assessments will help you discover whether your
constitution is balanced, Cold or Hot, Damp or Dry, weak or strong,
or perhaps even a combination. Once you know your constitution,
it will help you choose, with this book as a guide, the correct
ingredients to achieve a balance of Yin and Yang. For instance, if
you have a Dry constitution, select black sesame and wolfberries
as cooling and neutral nourishment. However, you must be careful
not to consume too much or for too long, or it might make your
constitution overly Damp.

Another approach to choosing food is to do so according to the
organs and related meridians. If you have a Dry constitution, the
reason could be Dryness in the lung or kidney. For Dryness in the
kidney, you would again use wolfberries and black sesame. However
for Dryness in the lung, lily bulbs or almonds are recommended. To
maximize the benefits, these ingredients should be used for at least
one month. Food therapy is based on the generalized constitution
combined with individual needs. Once you have achieved the right
balance, you can once again enjoy a broad diet.

To achieve balance and longevity, it is paramount to understand
one's constitution and the factors that influence it. The basis of
TCM is rooted in this understanding, which is then used to create
treatment plans that will bring one's health to an optimal level.
These highly individualized remedies include changing lifestyle
habits and diet and taking supplements.

A person must understand his or her own constitution in order
to take the right steps to achieve good health. The assessments
below will help you learn more about your own constitution in order
to choose foods and herbs, health care methods, and lifestyle habits
specifically suited to your individual needs.

1. Questions Relating to Temperature: Neutral, Cold, Hot, or Mixed Constitution

Are you sensitive to the cold or heat?
- ☐ normal (1)
- ☐ sensitive to cold (2)
- ☐ sensitive to heat (3)

What do you prefer to drink?
- ☐ depends on season (1)
- ☐ warm/hot drinks (2)
- ☐ cold drinks (3)

Do you sweat a lot?
- ☐ normal (1)
- ☐ less than average (2)
- ☐ more than average (3)

How do you classify your thirst?
- ☐ normal (1)
- ☐ not often thirsty (2)
- ☐ often thirsty (3)

How is your complexion?
- ☐ shining and rosy (1)
- ☐ pale and puffy (2)
- ☐ flushed (3)

How is your tongue coating when you get up in the morning?
- ☐ thin white coating (1)
- ☐ thick white coating (2)
- ☐ thick yellow coating (3)

What is your pulse (beats per minute)?
- ☐ from 60 to 80 (1)
- ☐ less than 60 (2)
- ☐ over 80 (3)

How often do you drink tea or coffee?
- ☐ up to two cups of coffee or tea everyday (1)
- ☐ three or more cups of tea everyday (2)

☐ three or more cups of coffee everyday (3)

What kind of food do you prefer?
☐ depends on season (1)
☐ a light taste or raw food (2)
☐ spicy or strongly flavored food (3)

Assessment:
Neutral: 6 or more responses of (1)
Cold: 6 or more of (2)
Hot: 6 of more of (3)
Mixed: if fewer than 6 of
any one response

Cold or Hot constitution.

2. Questions Relating to Humidity: Neutral, Damp, Dry, or Mixed Constitution

What is your tongue like?
☐ normal size with a thin white coating (1)
☐ large with a thick or wet coating (2)
☐ small with a thin or dry coating (3)

What kind of taste do you usually have in your mouth?
☐ normal (1)
☐ sticky and sweet (2)
☐ dry (3)

What is your skin condition?
☐ normal or mixed (1)
☐ oily (2)
☐ dry or cracking (3)

How would you characterize your excretion? (Discharge from eyes, ears and skin; for women, including monthly period)
☐ comfortable amount (1)
☐ quite a lot (2)
☐ scant or absent (3)

Do you smoke or drink alcohol?
☐ occasionally (1)
☐ frequently (2)

☐ refrain from both (3)

What is your tolerance for dairy products?
☐ average (1)
☐ less than average (2)
☐ more than average (3)

How do you feel in general?
☐ happy and relaxed (1)
☐ heavy, sleepy, fullness in chest and stomach (2)
☐ irritable, anxious, dry lips and throat (3)

How would you characterize your bowel movements and urine output?
☐ normal (1)
☐ loose stool or turbid urine (2)
☐ dry stool, constipation or scanty urine (3)

How would you describe your build?
☐ average (1)
☐ heavy build (2)
☐ slim (3)

Damp or Dry constitution.

Assessment:
Neutral: 6 or more responses of (1)
Damp: 6 or more of (2)
Dry: 6 or more of (3)
Mixed: if fewer than 6 of any one response

3. Questions Regarding Your Response to Adversity: Neutral, Weak, Overly Strong, or Mixed Constitution

Do you feel energetic?
☐ average (1)
☐ more than average (2)
☐ less than average (3)

What is your tongue like when you get up in the morning?
☐ pink body and thin coating (1)
☐ dark or purple body and thick coating (2)
☐ pale or deeper red body and no coating (3)

What kind of food do you prefer?
☐ mixed, with more vegetables and less meat (1)
☐ mostly meat (2)
☐ vegetarian (3)

How often is your elimination?
☐ normal (1)
☐ infrequent (2)
☐ too frequent (3)

How often do you get a cold every year?
☐ once or few times (1)
☐ never (2)
☐ often (3)

How often do you get excited?
☐ normal (1)
☐ frequently (2)
☐ seldom (3)

How do your muscles feel?
☐ normal (1)
☐ tight and sore (2)
☐ soft and weak (3)

How quickly do you feel shortness of breath when hiking?
☐ 15 minutes to half an hour (1)
☐ more than half an hour (2)
☐ after a few minutes (3)

How does your head often feel?
☐ normal (1)
☐ pressure or sharp headache (2)
☐ lightheaded or dizziness (3)

Assessment:
Neutral: 6 or more responses of (1)
Overly Strong: 6 or more of (2)
Weak: 6 or more of (3)
Mixed: if fewer than 6 of any one response

Weak or overly strong constitution.

In completing the above self-assessment, we encountered some pairs of concepts, such as Cold or Hot, Damp or Dry, and overly strong or weak. All these feelings, when within a certain range, are normal for us to feel. We should feel cold in winter and hot in summer. However, if we always feel cold, even in spring, or feel cold too often, then we should seek the underlying reason and try to remedy it.

The approach toward Damp and Dry is similar. Both are necessary and normal within boundaries. Dampness nourishes our inside and moistens the surface of the skin, while Dryness limits the growth of mold. However, too much Dampness makes skin oily and prone to acne. In turn, too much Dryness brings wrinkles and cracking. Therefore, we should stay Neutral as long as we can.

Now that you have assessed your constitution, we can use that information to choose the right foods and herbs to help you achieve and maintain balance.

Let's take the Damp, Dry, and Neutral constitution as an example. If you have a Neutral type, it means you are quite balanced. In order to keep this state, it is best to eat a broad range of foods and be sure to drink water according to the climate and your level of perspiration. However, if you have a Damp constitution, this means there is too much humidity inside of you. You need to add specific foods to your diet (such as pearl barley, red beans, corn, or winter squash) to reduce Dampness and bring yourself back to balance. A Dry type, on the other hand, would have different requirements for a healthy diet. In this case, foods such as lily bulb, wolfberry, honey, or lemon can nourish and moisten the body.

Chapter Seven
Why Do We Become Sick

In this chapter we will talk about the causes of disease (the pathogeny).

Previously, we introduced different concepts regarding healthy body conditions, especially the balance between Yin and Yang, the balance between mental activity and physical function, and the balance between the meridians and the five organ systems. If there is disharmony between any external and internal factors, harming the balance in our body or breaking down the equilibrium between the body and the environment, this imbalance will cause the body to transit from being in a healthy condition to a sub-healthy condition, and it could eventually lead to certain diseases. The study of the causes, from external to internal, that could lead to disease is called etiology.

According to TCM, the cause of disease can be divided into two categories. The first category is our external environment, including change of weather, seasons, and geographic conditions. The second category is the internal body, especially focusing on our lifestyle, how we deal with our food, and our emotional state. In this sense, as you can see, most of the TCM ideas related to the cause of a disease are tied to our basic environment, such as the current weather, location we live and work, our constitution, how we deal with our emotions, and how we choose and eat our food.

External Causes of a Disease

External causes of disease in TCM are divided into two parts:
- Six excessive climatic factors (*liu yin*), referring to excessive Wind, Coldness, Summer-Heat, Dampness (humidity), Dryness, and Fire (heat).
- Epidemic factors (*li qi*), referring to highly contagious, transmissible diseases, which we will not address in this book.

Wind, Coldness, Summer-Heat, Dampness (humidity), Dryness, and Fire (heat) are six kinds of natural climatic factors known as *liu qi*. Each dominates during a different season.

In winter, Coldness will be predominant. In summer, Summer-Heat will be predominant. They change with each season, and they are very important climate types for the growth and development of plants, humans, and other creatures. For example, in the five elements, most species wake up in the spring time, sprout, garner new life, then quickly grow during summer and transform during the humid season (plum rain season in Asia), are harvested in autumn, and store energy in winter. This kind of change can be combined with the six climatic factors as well. Generally speaking, the six climatic factors do not disturb our health and wellbeing because most human beings and plants, through evolution, are equipped to adapt to different changes. There are only three reasons that can cause the six climates (*liu qi*) to change to six excessive climatic factors (*liu yin*).

The first reason is extreme climate/weather. For example, in Shanghai, the temperature during summer usually ranges between 30 and 38 degrees celsius. If the heat increases one summer to reach 42 or 45 degrees celsius, it could lead to people suffering from heat stroke (*zhong shu*) or other types of illness. The second reason is sudden changes in the weather. For example, during winter, starting from December and ending around February, we should have a temperature range between -2 and 5 degrees celsius. If winter temperatures suddenly change to 15 degrees, it could also cause people difficulty in adapting and cause flu or certain digestive maladies. The third reason is not external but internal, referring to people having a weak body constitution. This would create problems in dealing with different external climate factors.

Now we understand that changes in temperature and humidity can change many organisms and microbes in the biosphere in which we live. Wind, Coldness, and so forth are terms for groups of symptoms. Modern research shows Wind, Coldness, Fire, and Dampness are actually various meteorological and biological pathogenic factors that act in synthesis to create various symptoms manifested by the human body.

Therefore, compared with the viral and bacterial causes mentioned in the biological etiology of modern medicine, TCM etiology takes into account that there are more subtypes of human responsiveness. The combination of the two can ensure more accurate diagnosis and treatment.

The above reasons explain how the six climates can change to six excessive climatic factors. We can summarize the six excessive climatic/pathogenic factors into four common characteristics.

First, they disturb us by entering our body through the skin, nose, or mouth. For instance, during springtime, many people will suffer from flu or hepatitis A. This is usually caused by Wind combined with Heat entering our body through the nose and mouth.

Second, they are usually related to the seasons and the patient's environment. During autumn, the predominant factor is Dryness, and that can easily invade the lungs to cause seasonal bronchitis. During long winter, people living in northern parts of the city or certain geographical environments might have more cold patterns invading their systems. The pathogenic factors relate to the seasons and our environment.

Third, they can transform after invading the body. When the Coldness factor enters our body, it can change into Heat. The pathogenic factors don't change, but our body's constitution can change the different factors and therefore the pattern. For example, a person with Dampness can transform Heat into Heat Dampness. Even if the season is not that humid, people might show Dampness in their body.

Fourth, they can attack the body individually or in combination. For instance, Wind can enter our body by itself to cause Wind patterns, just as Coldness or Heat can. But many times they also attack in combination. Let's take arthritis for example. TCM refers to arthritis as a *bi* (pain or numbness) syndrome. When people suffer from this syndrome, the type of aching or pain might be in joints, lower back, or certain muscles. The combination will be Wind, Dampness, and Coldness, three excessive climatic factors coming together. We have to identify which is predominant. If Wind is predominant, we need to treat Wind first, and Dampness and Coldness will follow. Clinically, we call Wind-predominant syndromes wandering-*bi* syndromes, because the pain is not fixed and it can move freely and quickly from different body parts, shoulder to knees to hips. Simple exercise can help to minimize the pain. Generally, when we treat this, we have to use the expelling method to open skin pores, letting the Wind come out from the body. If Coldness is predominant, we call it Cold *bi*. This manifestation is more fixed pain all the time, such as a fixed shoulder pain. Cold temperatures can make it worse. Sometimes when the pain is too extreme, the patient may need painkillers. We call this painful *bi*. Warm methods can help relieve pain temporarily. For example people moving to warm areas/climates, putting more clothes on, going to the sauna or using warm patches or heating bags filled with beans to give warmth to painful areas can provide some relief. When Dampness is predominant, we call it Damp *bi*. People will not just feel joint pain but will also feel a heaviness,

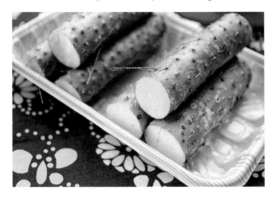

Chinese yam.

swelling, and fullness inside. Often, people describe this feeling as soreness rather than pain. To treat this, we must use methods to remove Dampness. For example, many people add pearl barley or barley to their diet, or Chinese yam to help tone their energy and strengthen their energy flow to remove the Dampness. This explains how climatic factors can affect people in combination, but you still need to identify which is predominant.

Now we will introduce each excessive climatic/pathogenic factor one by one.

1. Wind 风

Wind is more related to the spring season, and it is more associated with the liver system. The three major features when it comes to causing disease are:

Wind is a Yang factor, light and opening. It moves very fast (think tornado) and when our skin pores and orifices are open, will feel aversion to Wind and easily sweat.

Wind moves upwards and outwards. It easily rises up and affects the upper portion of the body, including the head and face. Itchiness in the eyes and nose causing people to rub their eyes or sneeze usually indicates Wind rising. Could even cause facial paralysis, such as deviances or spasms in the mouth and eyes.

Wind can easily cause change. It is not usually a fixed pain. For instance, certain skin rashes caused by Wind can move from different parts of your body, from behind the ears to above the eyes. The location migrates. Also, it can easily open the door to let other pathogens enter and even transform and cause other diseases. The form of the pattern can vary. Wind combined with Dampness can cause more of a runny nose or teary eyes. If Wind is not combined with any other pathogens, it can enter and affect the body quickly, but also leave it quickly, but if it is combined with Dampness or Coldness, it can take much longer to treat it.

2. Coldness 寒

Coldness is more related to the winter season and the kidney system.

Coldness can be constricting, causing rigid tendons and tight blood vessels. Frozen shoulder, for example, is caused by excess Coldness. Skin pores are also constricted, therefore causing a lack of sweat. If a person sleeping in bed is rolled up like a ball, they are more affected by Coldness. This is how doctors have traditionally diagnosed patients. If they sleep sprawled out, that usually indicates that they are affected by Heat.

Coldness is an Yin factor. Many people who are affected have cold hands and feet and start to feel cold in autumn. They have an aversion to cold, and usually when this pattern starts they have no sweat (as opposed to the Wind pattern, which will cause sweat). It can also damage the body's Yang energy, making energy move slowly and eventually weakening.

Coldness can block and obstruct, including stagnating Qi and Blood, causing symptoms of aching and pain. This is induced by cold environments and climates or personal preferences, such as drinking cold beverages or foods with Cold properties (for instance, white meat, like seafood is more Cold than red meat). Tendons and meridian channels can also be blocked and obstructed.

3. Summer-Heat 暑

Summer-heat is related to the summer season and to the heart system. It is specific to periods from the 24 solar terms, from summer solstice, usually around June 21, to the beginning of autumn, usually around August 8. Any similar patterns during the rest of the year would be categorized as Fire (heat).

Summer-Heat is a Yang factor. Excess Yang & Heat go upwards, disturbing the mind. It splits into two kinds. One is Heat disturbing our temperature center (heat stroke), which can be treated by moving to colder places or drinking cooling beverages. Another is more infectious Heat that can injure the body system, causing high fever, thirst, perspiration, constipation, distraction, and delirium. This requires comprehensive treatment, as it could be a virus or bacterial infection.

Summer-Heat, like Wind, also moves in an outward motion, so it can cause excess sweating. Excess sweat can cause exhaustion of the body energy and dehydration. To control Summer-Heat, it is important to ensure body liquids with proper hydration. The symptoms of energy weakness are shortness of breath, fatigue, and lethargy. The symptoms of dehydration are dry lips, throat, and mouth and drinking liquids but not quenching thirst. Especially for vegetarians, eating more summer berries, root vegetables, and beans (such as mung bean soup) can help with protecting Body Fluids and toning Qi.

If there is a rainy season before or after the summer season (for example, in Shanghai, it is in June and July), many times Summer-Heat symptoms can be combined with Dampness. The symptoms can change. For example, if combined with Dampness, the fever might not be too high. If there is only Summer-Heat, there might be excess perspiration, but with Dampness, there will be less perspiration, but stickier. There will be more symptoms related to Dampness, which you will see in the next section. If combined with Dampness, it requires different herbs or treatments to control both symptoms.

4. Dampness 湿

Dampness is more related to a rainy season, a geographical area with more humidity, or a working environment that has more contact with water (fishermen for example). It is related to the spleen system.

Coldness and Dampness are both Yin factors, but Coldness invades the body more easily and damages the Yang energy. Dampness has more visible factors, which can include water or mucus trapped in the body. It will cause Yang energy to stagnate, then cause it to weaken, but it takes time and is not as strong as Coldness.

If Dampness invades the body, you will feel heavy and turbid in the muscles and limbs. Excretion from the body's sensory organs, such as the throat, ears, eyes, and nose, will be stickier with grey, yellow, or green colors. For example, ear infections will have yellow mucus, and urinary tract/kidney infections combined with Dampness will result in cloudy urine (too much protein in the urine). Even sweat can be sticky with a foul odor.

Dampness can make certain illnesses last longer compared to other pathogens and take a longer time to be cured. For example, arthritis, asthma, and eczema or other acute infections combined with Dampness require a longer treatment and recovery period.

Dampness moves downward. It is Yin, which is shaped more like water, therefore its features/nature is more like water, more easily disturbed in the areas below the waist, especially causing joint swelling, diarrhea, irregular female vaginal discharge, and skin conditions in groin area. In TCM, the area above the waist is more Yang and that below the waist is Yin. Wind relates to more of the upper body, head, and back area, whereas Dampness correlates more with bottom half of the body.

5. Dryness 燥
Dryness is associated with the autumn season and is linked to the lung system.

Dryness tends to impair Body Fluids and energy. Symptoms can include dry mouth, throat, and nose, skin cracks in the hands and feet, dry cough, or sticky mucus with blood. It can cause flu, bronchitis, and throat infections due to a weakened immune system.

Dryness itself cannot be called a Yin or Yang factor, but its patterns can vary according to early or late autumn. During early autumn, there is leftover Summer-Heat, and the temperature is still relatively high, so the Dryness can be combined with Heat, a condition called Warm Dryness factor. When the Dryness is closer to winter, the Dryness can be combined with Coldness, forming Cool Dryness factor.

Dryness tends to impair the lung and stomach. According to TCM's understanding, the lung and stomach are the most delicate organs in terms of their need for moisture. Dryness can easily damage these two areas of the body, resulting in a dry cough, coughing sticky mucus with blood, thirst, and conditions of the lungs and surface of the skin. It must be prevented through drinking more juice from natural plants and vegetable soups.

6. Fire (Heat) 火
Like Summer-Heat, Fire (heat) is related to the heart system, and it is a Yang factor. However, it occurs during the period outside of Summer-Heat (between June 21st and August 8th). In TCM, there are varying degrees of this Heat. Warm is the lowest degree,

Heat is medium, and Fire is highest.

Fire is a Yang factor and moves in an outward motion (refer to the same features of Summer-Heat on pages 78 and 79). Fire (heat) will induce Wind in the body and attack it rapidly. It can attack the liver, then quickly change/transform to another meridian or system. It can also increase blood circulation and cause bleeding. Symptoms also include involuntary spasms.

Fire (heat) tends to burn and scorch. When Fire makes the energy and blood stagnate and accumulate in a particular area, it can burn the muscles and cause sores, styes, and other skin discomfort. However, these skin problems can also be caused when touched by dirty hands.

These are how the six climates can change to become six excessive climatic/pathogenic factors.

Six Excess Climatic Factors	Nature Features	Features of Illness According to TCM	Symptoms
Wind	Yang factor, going upwards and outwards, light & opening	disturb Yang part of body (head & skin), open skin pores	aversion to wind, sweating, headache, upper back ache
	moveable, changeable, migrating	involuntarily moveable, location of symptoms migrate	itching, spasm, wandering joints ache, mouth and eyes deviate
	climate forerunner	combine Coldness, Heat, Dampness	have both Wind & Cold, Wind & Heat or Wind & Dampness symptom
Coldness	Yin factor	damage the body's Yang energy	aversion to cold, cold hands and feet
	blocking and obstructing	stagnate Qi and Blood of body	pain
	shrinking & constricting	Qi convergence & tight blood vessels, rigid tendons	no sweat, limited movement, contracture spine
Summer-Heat	Yang factor, excess Heat flames up	excess Yang & Heat disturb mind	high fevers, red face, distracted, delirious
	Heat outward	loss of liquid and good energy	sweat a lot, thirst, shortness of breath, fatigue
	Heat and humid	Dampness and Heat or Fire	sticky perspiration, heavy limbs and body muscles, fullness of chest

Dampness	Yin factor	stagnate Yang energy	poor appetite, soft stool, bloating & fullness
	heavy and turbid	visible substance, excretion grimy	heavy feeling of head & body, abnormal discharge from nose and eyes
	glued & obstructed	chronic & recurring	rheumatism, eczema
	heavy & downward bearing	disturb Yang part of body (below waist)	diarrhea, leucorrhea
Dryness	dry, withered	easily consume Body Fluid & Qi, disturb lung & stomach fluid	dry and crack skin, dry cough, thirst
Fire (Heat)	Yang factor, excess Heat flames up	excess Yang & Heat disturb mind	high fevers, red face, distracted, delirious
	Heat outward	loss of liquid and good energy	sweat a lot, thirst, shortness of breath, fatigue
	pressing	generate Wind & disturb Blood	involuntary spasm, bleeding, rapid pulse
	burning and scorching	block Qi & Blood, damage muscle & vessel	sores, styes, pimple and other skin agonies

Six excessive climatic factors.

Internal Impairment Due to the Seven Emotions

In the previous section we explored the exogenous causes of various ailments. Now let's learn about the internal causes of the disease. In TCM, most of the exogenous causes are acute, infectious diseases. With hepatitis A, what TCM calls the Damp-Heat type is just symbol of pathological conditions rather than real etiological factors. It comes from analysis of the whole picture of the body, including symptoms and signs.

Internal factors mainly cause chronic, recurrent diseases. Family hereditary disease, cardiac, cerebral arteriosclerosis, and other pathological changes, disorders of the endocrine system, low or hyper immune function, and other such conditions all belong to the category of diseases induced by internal causes.

TCM's theory of internal causes of pathogens includes emotional disorder, dietary imbalances, inappropriate work and rest balance, and other factors to make us unwell. Above all, it is related to our personality type (introverted, extroverted), how we respond to social factors, and our choice of foods and lifestyle. They should be normal parts of our life. Only when the symptoms become intense and the intense condition lasts for a prolonged period or our abilities to adapt to them decrease can they turn to internal causes of diseases. Now let's start with Seven Pathogenic Emotions.

1. Basic Theories and Viewpoints of Chinese Medicine Related to the Emotions

The seven emotions is a unique name TCM gives to the modern sense of emotion. It contains the main ideas found in modern emotional theory. The seven emotions refer to normal emotions of joy, anger, worry, thinking (longing), sadness, fear, and shock. These are the normal physiological and emotional characteristics of human beings. For example, when you receive good news, you should feel happy. If you do not feel joy, it is an unreasonable and unnatural phenomenon. When you face an important exam, you should feel stress or a little worry. If your expression shows no stress, it would be unusual. TCM believes that "the seven emotions are people's regulator." It is both an instinctive impulse and a behavioral expression. It is both a kind of experience and a reaction, and it is a compound state of all human beings. As a person's regulator, healthy people have emotional reactions. It is one of the signs of psychological wellbeing, and some emotional reactions can also improve health.

2. The Relationship between the Seven Emotions and Qi, Blood, and Viscera

Emotion has a significance positive impact on the balance of the body and the mind. If emotional activities can maintain stability, it is commendable. As long as it is within the scope of the "physiological threshold," it is not only harmless, but can buffer external stimuli and facilitate the peace of organ functions. By contrast, the lack of any kind of emotion is a manifestation of imperfect physical-mental function.

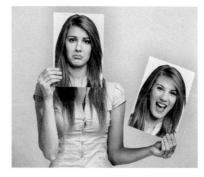

The seven emotions can be divided into Yin and Yang. Yang

The seven emotions are people's regulator.

refers to affirmation, positive emotions such as joy, and thinking. Yin refers to negativity, low emotions such as sadness, fear, and anger (easily combined with longing). We need both. The seven emotions are the types of emotions that the human body inherited genetically. They have two basic characteristics of biology and pathology, benign orientation and non-benign orientation, and two-level duality. TCM believes that the seven emotions are born in the viscera, out of the heart and brain, and are the expression of the unity of the body, mind, and emotions. "People have five organs and corresponding five Qi, and they are born with joy, sorrow, and fear." The physiology of the seven emotions refers to human reflection on the subjective and objective world, which is a normal spiritual activity. The seven emotions are the combination of biology, psychology, medical science, and other aspects.

Change in the seven emotions has a counter-effect on the human body, which can cause diseases under certain conditions. As a cause, the seven emotions refer to emotional stimulation acting on the human body suddenly, strongly, repeatedly, or permanently, exceeding the scope of the body's resistance or self-regulation, leading to visceral Qi dysfunction and causing mental or physical diseases. If the Qi and Blood of organs changes abnormally, it can also affect emotional activity. "The deficiency of liver Qi may cause a state of fear, but its excess may cause a state of anger." Thus the emotions can not only cause disharmony, but they can also be caused by it.

3. The Pathogenic Features of the Seven Pathogenic Emotions Directly Impair the Viscera

When all different emotions become causative factors, it usually starts from disharmony of the heart, then affects the corresponding viscera.

Over emotion harms the five internal organs. The general law is too much worry or sadness blocks or consumes the lung Qi, over fear make kidney Qi sink and descend, too much anger makes the liver Qi inversion heighten, excessive and sudden

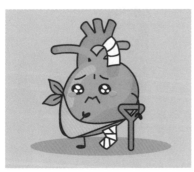

Over emotion harms internal organs.

joyful news make heart Qi out of order, and excess pensiveness stagnates the spleen Qi. TCM holds that human mental activities are closely related with the internal organs. The Chinese medical classic *Basic Questions* says, "Man has five viscera which may bring on five moods, producing joy, anger, sadness, pensiveness, and fear." It believes that certain viscera are related to certain emotional activities, i.e., the heart is related to joy, the liver to anger, the spleen to pensiveness, the lungs to sadness, and the kidney to fear.

The symptom of the emotional disorder shows more in the heart, liver, and spleen systems. TCM holds that mental activities need sufficient blood and good blood circulation, which are particularly related to the heart, liver, and spleen system. Clinical manifestations like insomnia, heart palpitations, dream disturbed sleep, forgetfulness, and madness are associated with the heart system.

Plum core throat (a feeling of obstruction in the pharynx, like there's a plum core in the throat, but without an organic lesion. It is caused mainly by upward inversion of stagnated liver Qi due to a poor mood), rib cage pain, menopause, premenstrual tension syndrome, and other conditions are associated with the liver system. Anger, an emotion belongs to Yang, lets people know your limits of interpersonal distance. When one accumulates or has excess anger, body energy flows up to disturb the upper portion of the body, for instance the neck and the side or top of the head.

Excessive pensiveness, neurasthenia, chronic diarrhea, stomach ulcers, upper gastrointestinal bleeding, and other symptoms are associated with the spleen system. Excess pensiveness or longing (having a crush on someone or something) blocks the spleen Qi's movement and affect digestion and absorption of nutrition. Workaholism, excessive cravings for sugar, and drinking too much coffee and wine could be harmful to the digestive system.

Influence the movements of Qi of the viscera. Excessive seven emotions influence the movements of the Qi through the organs. The disorder of the Qi can indicate Qi weakness. The speed of the Qi's movement becomes fast or slow or normal direction of the Qi movement runs into the opposite direction.

Which internal organ do harmful emotions affect? It's relative and varies from person to person. The examples listed here occur at a higher frequency. For instance, anger not only hurts the liver, but in different physiques and individuals, it can also do damage to the heart or the kidney. In the end, in noting which viscera are affected, it is necessary to consider all the symptoms and signs of the patient. In the case of a small number of accompanying symptoms, it can be prioritized according to one of our five elements pairings.

For example, happiness is an emotion that belongs to the Yang. It can relax the whole body and harmonize the internal system. But excessive excitement and sudden joyful news can disturb the movement order of the heart Qi, especially attacking stressed and weak people.

Excessive happiness is possible when coming into new fortune. How many times do we hear of people fainting when winning the lottery or hitting the jackpot? Those with a strong constitution whose emotions are less strong and who can handle these emotions can face it with grace, but those with a fickle constitution are usually affected more easily.

Tending to cause mental disease and psychosomatic disorder. The seven pathogenic emotions frequently induce psychosomatic disorder and mental and emotional illness, such as IBS, epilepsy, and psychosis. The changes and the trends of the disease are closely related to the emotions. They can aggravate or worsen if the emotional state is poor. One of my clients has a family history of high cholesterol and hypertension. During his 40's, his cholesterol level broke through normal values. One day he was very stressed and angry while managing a project meeting. During discussion, he got angry about some points. His face turned red, his head hurt, and the right side of his body grew numb. His colleague took him to the hospital for an examination and found that his blood pressure was high and he had a cerebral vasospasm. After treatment, his physical condition recovered. The doctor's advice was to decrease and avoid anger and losing his temper. He learned from the case and became more active in moderate exercise, trying to improve his irritable personality.

Internal Impairment Due to Dietary Disorders

The second means of determining the internal cause of a disease is to explore the endogenous dietary factors.

Medicine and foods are homologous. It is advisable to eliminate wrong eating habits, especially dieting, skipping meals, or eating erratically, because they can lower blood sugar, causing symptoms such as weakness, irritability, and fatigue. We should make food easy to digest and suited to the individual, grasping the three principles of eating order, seasonable, balanced, and diverse. Take whole food, reduce unnecessary cooking and processing procedures, make various nutrients match each other, and use synergy and performance across the board so you can enjoy eating a rainbow of colors and richer tastes, taking the maximum amount of nutrition, fighting illness, and keeping fit!

There are three major beliefs about food in Chinese medicine:

Food is the cornerstone of life. It nourishes, provides vitamins and minerals, promotes growth, and enhances longevity. It is life-sustaining. Functional food can also help to prevent or treat certain illnesses.

Some foods can be harmful or cause illness. In some people or under certain conditions, foods can cause acute or immediate reactions and problems. Examples include allergies, food poisoning, and symptoms related to lactose intolerance. Timing and amount of food consumption can also negatively impact the digestive system, such as enduring prolonged hunger or long gaps between meals, or eating and drinking too much at one meal. Over-eating one type of food also has a negative effect. An example is a patient who exercises regularly and eats healthy in every way, including a heavily vegetable-based diet, except that she eats dark chocolate every day and is eventually diagnosed with high cholesterol.

Another time that food can cause harm is when people eat foods that don't agree with their body. As we know, TCM believes that individual bodies may be more inclined to Hot or Cold constitutions. Those who are on the Hot side may experience more constipation, heartburn, or mouth ulcers. If this is the case, they should avoid foods that raise the Heat in the body, such as spicy foods, coffee, or hot soups. By contrast, people who are in the Cold spectrum may have an upset stomach from drinking too many cold drinks, eating ice cream, and so on, and therefore they should avoid too much raw foods, especially in winter, or other cold foods that make them feel ill, even if they enjoy the flavor.

Try to avoid too little food or sticking to a few limited items in your diet, which can cause malnutrition, lack of blood function, and low immune cells, further inducing many other diseases, such as anemia and amenorrhea. Severe cases can cause anorexia.

To avoid excess eating of certain types of foods, you should be mindful of your flavor preferences or aversions. Continually eating from only one flavor group can negatively impact various organs. For example, eating only spicy foods can make you sweat too much and reduce water content in the body, making the lungs dry out. Likewise, too much salt can negatively impact the kidneys as they struggle to filter the body properly. People who eat many sweet things, such as cookies or anything with added sugar, will often face problems with their pancreas from over stimulation and too much insulin production and become overweight.

Undigested food becoming stagnant in the digestive tract can lead to chronic ailments. This may happen if food is not digested thoroughly, if it is not passed in a timely manner, or if particles become stuck in the intestines. Signs that food has accumulated in the digestive tract may include poor appetite, belching, gas with a distinct smell, bloating or diarrhea, and in severe cases, painful heartburn with a bitter taste in the throat and mouth. When not resolved, gastritis, irritable bowel syndrome (IBS), pancreatitis, and gallstones are likely to occur. Polyps can also develop in the colon, leading to colon cancer.

Foods and herbs have specific therapeutic actions beyond their temperature, color, and taste or the meridians traveled. A food may either tone/strengthen a particular substance or function (Qi, Blood, Yin and Yang), or it may reduce or regulate the influence of a pathological condition (Qi or Blood stagnation, Dampness, Heat or Coldness). Lychee, for example, reduces Coldness and regulates blood circulation to treat pigmentation on the face. Kidney bean tone the Yang.

Therefore, it is important to put all the qualities of food together to fully understand its therapeutic effect. For example, people with a Cold constitution can choose red wine or pomegranates, but they need to understand first that red wine enters all meridians, while pomegranate enters only the Lung, Kidney, and Large Intestine Meridians. Similarly, those with Hot constitutions might choose green tea, which enters the Heart, Stomach, and Kidney Meridians. Another choice is the blueberry, which enters the Lung, Spleen, and Stomach Meridians. Body constitution, food temperature and taste, and the meridians the food travels must be considered to choose the perfect food for you.

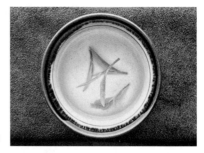

Green tea.

This tailor-made knowledge helps judge one's individual needs when choosing functional food, herbs, and supplements. There are so many choices out there, and decisions can often be made on superficial terms, influenced by packaging or advertising. However, if you understand the basics of Chinese medicine, your choices will be wiser, allowing foods to work holistically to help you get and stay healthy. (See more in Chapter Six to know your constitution.)

Internal Impairment Due to an Imbalanced Lifestyle

Lifestyle plays a big role in achieving the balance required for lasting health. We consider daily activities and habits, including work time and leisure time, as imperative to achieving social and mental well-being. It is essential to know how, when, and how to spend your energy.

In modern society, work often dictates how we spend the majority of our days for those who are employed. Those in knowledge-based jobs that require much mental work or who spend most of their time on tasks that require thinking, concentration, and focus may experience Blood and energy deficiencies. Similarly, those in jobs that require significant physical work, such as sports, manual labor, and outdoor activities may also experience a Qi deficiency.

Both types of work require achieving a balance to ensure that individuals do not do too much at one thing. These days, we see people labeled as "workaholics," many of whom experience "burnout" or "breakdowns" as a result of not being able to manage their time and energy.

The ways to achieve this balance vary between individuals, depending on their own levels of discipline, goals, and work styles, but ultimately everyone must find their own balance to ensure longevity and health.

If you are a freelancer, not working, or retired, you have much more control over your daily schedule, as you are not bound by office hours. It is therefore easier to live in accordance with the universe and follow the patterns of the sunrise and sunset each day. For optimal health, try to wake with the sun, eat three regularly spaced meals throughout the day, and go to bed after sunset. We should also follow the seasonal changes as a guide for each day. For example, during winter it is important to conserve energy. Go to bed earlier to retain Yang energy, and wait for sunrise to wake up in order to store more energy. In the summer, there will be more energy from the sun for activities throughout the day, where you can spend more energy and Essence on daily activities. In these summer months, go to bed later in accordance with the sun setting later and wake up earlier, when it gets light, adding in rest after lunch to boost body and mind.

Avoid too little motion, sitting and using your cell phone or watching television too much. TCM says *jiu wo shang qi*, which means sitting or lying too long will cause the muscles to shrink or atrophy and the energy movement to stagnate, gradually causing a lack of energy. Researchers at Columbia University followed more than 3,500 adults in Jackson, Mississippi, for an average of 8.5 years and concluded that compared with those who watched TV for less than two hours a day, those who sat and watched TV for more than four hours a day had a 50% increased risk of heart disease. Let's move and enjoy nature more.

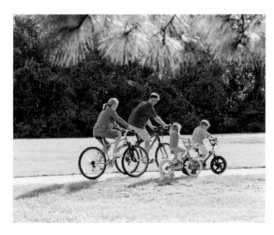

Move and enjoy nature more.

Chapter Eight
Catching Early Signals from Our Body

In Chinese medicine, we look at the various factors that can induce illness. They are often a result of our environment and our daily living conditions, including lifestyle, food, emotions, and spiritual elements.

To assess whether they are in balance, TCM looks for early

Traditional Chinese Medicine's General Diagnostic Procedures
There are many differences between patient diagnosis in TCM and the procedures used in Western medicine. The following is the general diagnostic procedure I use with TCM.

First, I examine the patient's physical build, facial complexion, and eyes. Then, I observe their posture while standing and sitting. I then speak with the patient, listening to the quality of their voice and trying to gauge the logic and speed of responses in conversation. Next, I look into the client's eyes to determine their brightness and shape, which relates to the health of their internal organs. Then I examine the tongue and the tongue's coating to understand the state of the patient's Qi and any invasive elements. Finally, I look under the tongue to check the flow of blood throughout the body.

Checking the patient's pulse is a vital part of this examination. With Western medicine, checking the pulse only entails counting the number of heartbeats per minute, but with TCM, we undertake a detailed evaluation of the heartbeat. I first take the Cun Guan Chi, or "Three Pulses," to determine the floating, middle, and deep level of meridian and organ energy flow. For example, in a normal pulse, my three fingers can feel the strength of the pulse on the middle level of energy flow. If I can only feel the pulse on a deep level with one or two fingers, there is most likely a problem.

It is also important to take note of the pulse's tempo. This indicates whether the blood flow has the right rhythm, which influences the fluctuations of a patient's mood. An even, steady beat equals an even, steady mood. Finally, I feel for the blood flow in the patient's veins, making sure that there is an adequate amount of blood and strong blood flow. Sometimes it is necessary to check both the left and right hands for a more thorough analysis.

signals from the body. We explain four different ways in which we can recognize signals of when the body is transitioning from healthy to unhealthy. The tools that can let us catch early onset information is called the "four methods of diagnosis." They are: looking (using the eyes); listening & smelling (using the ears & nose); asking (using the mouth); feeling or palpation (using the hands).

Looking

We can look at the whole body or a specific part of the body. For the whole body, TCM always looks at the tongue as a general indicator. If you have a problem in a certain area of the body, TCM will look at the specific part too. When we look at the whole body, we divide it into four parts.

First, we look at one's vitality or Spirit. The best way to understand this is through the eyes, facial expression, speech, and breathing. For example, if we look at the eyes, a TCM doctor considers looking at his/her Spirit. If the eyes are sparkling, glittering, and bright, this indicates a lively, energetic Spirit. Logical, clear speech and even breathing (16 to 18 breaths/min) shows a rich, healthy Spirit. This is also an indication of stable energy.

Lack of vitality can be seen through dull or cloudy eyes or lack of eye contact. Uncontrollable or blurred speech usually happens before one loses consciousness. Hyperthyroidism makes the eyeballs huge but dull and not shining, therefore a TCM doctor will suggest a thyroid check. If someone looks fatigued or lethargic or has a lack of focused response (confusion) or a low voice, it also indicates low levels of vitality and a weak Spirit. Breathing may also be uneven or short.

Second, we look at skin color and luster. Normal skin color

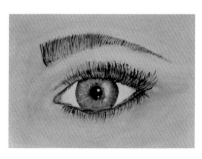

Eyes are the window of the soul.

and luster should be pink and representative of your nationality. (For example, for a Chinese person, it's pink-yellow, for Westerners it's pink-white, for African people it's pink-black). Luster should be glowing, clear, moist, and shining. Any change in the color would be an indication of illness. For example, redness or even purple in the face, spider veins on the cheek, or rosacea nose indicate menopause, heart problems, and alcoholism. Bacterial infection, allergy to dust mites, or accumulated toxins from over consumption of alcohol will cause redness, pimples, and an enlarged red nose. If yellow is present in the eyes or face, it may indicate jaundice. If a light yellow face looks anaemic with puffiness, it indicates weakness of Blood. If the skin underneath the eyes is black, it points to issues with sleep or the reproductive system. It could also be pigmentation, a blood circulation issue. If there's black around the mouth, one needs to do further investigation, as it shows something happening inside the body. If there is color change, also with no shine, or dry peeling skin, such as cracked hands or feet, then one would need to see a doctor to do some physical examination.

Third, we look at the patient's build and posture. If they have a large build and have recently experienced significant weight gain that they cannot lose weight through changes in diet and exercise, we may need to check their thyroid and adrenal function. Sugar intolerance, insulin resistance, or lowered energy levels could be preventing them from maintaining regular metabolism. If they have a slight built and are still losing weight, on the other hand, this indicates that the patient could be suffering from malnourishment, Blood deficiency, or digestive problems, that the blood circulation becomes blocked, or that the body has built up inner Fire.

Posture is also a way of judging a person's Yin/Yang constitution. If a person's posture is straight as a tree trunk while seated, and when they lie down their body remains open, this is more of a Yang person. If while sitting a person maintains a posture that is curved like a ball, and their body shrinks in size when they lie down, this indicates that they are more of a Yin person.

Fourth, one's movements show if he/she is Yang or Yin. If he/she walks with straight posture and with confident movement, then he/she is Yang. If he/she lacks energy and the movements are slow, then he/she is Yin.

In addition, we look at the condition of a person's tongue.

Tongue body. The normal color of the tongue is pink and bright, and it should be moist. The tongue should be not too big or small. There is small space between the corners of the mouth when we stick out our tongue. Whether the size of the tongue is normal,

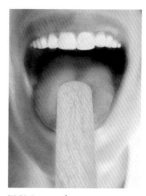

TCM uses the tongue as a key indicator of health.

big or small depends on the proportion of the tongue to the head, as well as the ratio of the tongue to the head and the whole body.

Tongue coating. The normal coating is thin and white, spreading evenly, and very moist.

Tongue movement. It should be able to move freely, should be able to move in all directions. When you stick out your tongue, its position is in the center.

There is a health care method that involves exercising the tongue's movement. Let your tongue roll and touch each corner of the gums. After 3 to 5 minutes, this will generate much saliva, which is healthy for nourishing the mouth, like a mouth wash. When we practice Qigong or meditation, our mouth, especially underneath the tongue, generates Body Fluids and helps the body relax and gain strength and flexibility. Swallowing the saliva will nourish the inside of the body.

If there is a change in the tongue from its normal condition, we should investigate and make some changes. Let's explain the different changes which are related to the tongue body and tongue coating.

Tongue body color change. If the tongue body changes from pink to other colors, we need to take a closer look. However, be mindful that it can be changed by food, and this should be excluded. The best time to look at your tongue is early morning after you wake up and before you drink anything.

If it is purple, there is stagnation of the Blood, which can be shown by purple dots around the edge or the whole tongue body appearing purple. When you check underneath, if the two veins are enlarged or are dark purple, this indicates that you need more blood circulation and an increase of food such as turmeric or an increase in water intake. The solution is dependent on your daily lifestyle. For example, if you already drink a lot of water, you may need to add food to help bring the liquid to the Blood. Some people may need exercise, usually outdoor exercise.

If the color is pale, it indicates a weak or Cold person. We should start with a warm drink and warm breakfast. Some cases may be combined with low body temperature and low blood pressure.

If the color is red or deep red, it indicates a Hot constitution. The patient's body needs a lot of liquid, and water is not spread evenly, accumulating in certain parts of the body and leaving other parts dry. Room temperature water in the morning, vegetables, and good oils from seeds or nuts will make the Body Fluid spread more evenly and nourish the body.

Tongue shape change. If the shape changes from normal to thin and small, it means the body is Hot or dehydrated. If your body Heat becomes excessive, you need to increase Cool food. If you lack Body Fluid, then strengthen body liquids. For example, increase consumption of mint tea to cool your body, or flaxseed to moist and nourish the body.

This will generate more moisture, and the tongue will not be thin or limp. If the tongue becomes bigger and thicker and has tooth marks, it indicates energy or Yang deficiency and water retention. A warm wholegrain breakfast will rebuild energy in the morning, such as oats, quinoa, or glutinous black rice. You should add Warm food such as cinnamon, mustard, and leeks. You can also try stretching and opening your spine, which helps energy move to the top of the body.

Tongue coating change. If the color changes from white to yellow, this indicates Heat inside the body (excluding situations in which you have eaten or drunk orange or carrot juice), so you need to eat cooling food such as cabbage and celery. If the color is white and thick, or if the saliva becomes sticky, it usually indicates Coldness inside the body. It is indicative of problems in the digestive system, often after using antibiotics. There could also be gas, bloating, and discomfort in the intestine. You can eat some Warm foods such as grains or mustard root to stimulate energy and remove water and Dampness. If the color is gray or dark, even nearly black, then you need to go to see a doctor. This is often seen in people who have smoked for a long time. If the tongue texture is wet and thick, it shows accumulated Dampness and water retention. A thin, dry tongue indicates excess Heat and a deficiency of Body Fluids.

Tongue movement change. It can indicate the early stage of certain diseases, such as central nervous system changes, including the early stages of stroke. If the tongue points to one side rather than the center, the central nervous system (CNS) is disturbed. If it is combined with a high fever of 42 to 43 degree celsius, the tongue may be trembling, indicating spasms in the upper body, such as the neck. You need to immediately lower the temperature, as this can cause damage to the CNS, which can lead to permanent damage. Once the temperature lowers down to 37 to 38 degree celsius, it is safe. If the tongue is on one side and a virus affects the facial nerves, it can lead to facial paralysis.

Listening and Smelling

We listen to different sounds, such as voice, speech, respiration, coughing, hiccups, or burping, to identify conditions.

If our voice has a high pitch and high volume, it usually indicates Heat or excess Yang condition. If the voice is low in volume and of a lower pitch, it usually indicates a weak, Cold, Yin condition. When we listen to a speech, if it is quick, clear, and fluent, there is an excess of Yang. If speech becomes weak, slow, and intermittent, this usually indicates an Yin condition, weak vitality, and Cold mental blockage. Where the respiration rate is too fast, from 18 to 25 breaths per minute, the heartbeat is also fast. This is indicative of a Hot, excess Yang condition, often combined with fever. When respiration becomes slow, combined with a slowing of the heartbeat or intermittent respiration, it is usually an Yin condition with Coldness or Phlegm blockage. Elderly people need to investigate more specifically to remove mucus and prevent the breathing from getting worse. Coughing is also an indicator, which can be dry or productive. When mucus came with a productive cough in ancient times, they would smell and examine the phlegm to determine the condition. A strong smell with a yellow green color indicated an excess. If there was a dry, intermittent cough, it could be Body Fluid deficiency or Qi deficiency. Tuberculosis is an example that presents with this type of cough. An asthmatic cough combined with heavy mucus and a wheezing sound, where the mucus is white, indicates an excess Cold Damp syndrome.

If there is excessive belching, hiccups, or acid reflux, it indicates a problem with the stomach and esophagus. If you feel relief after belching and the sound is loud, this is excess Qi. If the sound is weak and you feel no relief, it indicates a weakness of Qi. Hiccups come from diaphragm spasms and can be caused by eating food that is too dry or eating too fast. It can be remedied by drinking water, controlling the breathing, and raising your upper limbs. If the hiccups continue for a whole day, it can be indicative that a virus has invaded the diaphragm. If you have had an operation on the stomach, prolonged hiccuping can indicated that the digestive system is disturbed and needs to be addressed.

Smell from sweat, stool, and urine can also indicate some problems inside the body. A strong smell usually indicates an excess, while no smell or a light smell points to a deficiency. We can also check colors to identify a Cold or Hot constitution. Yellow, black, green, or bloody stool indicates Heat and Yin deficiency. White or transparent and watery stool indicates Yang deficiency and excess Coldness in body.

Asking

A TCM doctor will ask about 10 areas:

• Do you prefer hot or cold (climate, food, geographic location, etc)?

• How much do you sweat? How often? How quick? Spontaneous sweat shows a weakness of body energy, so you need to increase Qi from food. If we have night sweats, we need to increase Body Fluids.

• Do you have enough mental and physical energy? Do you prefer more mental work or more physical activity? How is your concentration and memory? If heart Qi, Blood, and spleen Qi are sufficient, you will think clearly and be able to concentrate and memorize things easily.

• Do you have aches and pains anywhere in the body? Aches and pains are meridian blockages. For example a stomachache can be Cold or Hot, so it is important to determine what causes it in order to diagnose the correct food to address it.

• How much do you sleep and how is the quality of the sleep? Normal sleep is between 6 to 8 hours without waking more than once. One should fall asleep quite quickly, in 15 to 30 minutes, and wake up feeling refreshed. If any of these areas are disturbed, i.e., not falling asleep, waking up many times, sleepwalking, or nightmares, then you need to identify the symptoms to determine whether the constitution is Hot or Cold and where there is weakness or excess.

• Identify your typical diet, tastes, and drink preference. TCM encourages a diet with a wide variety, based on local and seasonal foods. The motto is "eat the rainbow." This type of diet should provide us with most nutrients, so that we don't need supplements. Taste can indicate internal problems. For example, bitter taste after breakfast can indicate acid reflux, while a bitter taste all day can point to bacteria in the stomach (such as helicobacter pylori). A sweet taste all day can be a sign of Dampness. If you feel thirsty all the time and want to drink lots of water, it can show Dryness and weakness of Body Fluids. If you never feel thirsty or want to drink, you may have a blockage and mucus stagnation.

• Examine elimination and urination patterns. If you suffer from constipation, you are more Dry and Hot. If you have soft stool or diarrhoea, then you have more Coldness and weakness. If you have a lack of urine, it could be dehydration, indicating that you should drink more water. If you drink a normal amount of water but have infrequent urination, it could indicate serious kidney problems. For example, it can be an obstruction of the vesical calculi. If people drink a normal amount and urinate frequently, this may be a problem in the kidneys or bladder, or a urinary tract infection. If there's no pain or aches, it demonstrates a weak function of the kidneys and a need to strengthen the Blood in the urinary system and take kidney tonic foods, such as walnuts and kidney beans. If you are in pain, it's probably a urinary tract infection or bladder infection, which may require antibiotics.

• We must also take note of menstruation and vaginal

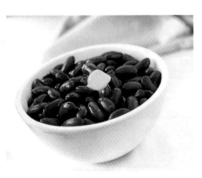

discharge. If you start menstruation on time (14 to 16 years), it is normal. During ovulation you can have a vaginal discharge similar to egg white. If the discharge becomes red or yellow, then a Hot condition is disturbing the reproductive organs. If there is a very watery or sticky white mucus, this could be due to Dampness and spleen

Kidney beans.

weakness.

• Childbirth, breastfeeding and infant disease are also important considerations. Was childbirth near to due time or very early? If it was very early, it indicates weakness. We recommend new mothers breastfeed their babies for about six months. If they go straight to formula or shorten the duration of breastfeeding, the child is more likely to develop allergies. How often does the child has flu/fever/ diarrhoea after breastfeeding? If it is more than three times per year, then he/she needs to strengthen the digestive and lung systems to develop a better constitution.

• Past history and family history is also important. We will ask about heart issues, high cholesterol, high lipids, diabetes, or cancer, especially breast, digestive, and colon cancer, in the family. If one is older, we will inquire about previous medical history to judge how much regulation and strengthening is needed for certain conditions.

Feeling or Palpation

Based on TCM's holistic approach, we use feeling to form a complete understanding of the person. By using all four methods together, we can obtain an overall picture of physical and mental health and be able to give appropriate advice. Feeling can be divided into two types. First, we consider the limbs, especially the surface of the skin. Second, we use pulse diagnosis.

1. Feeling of Limbs

In TCM, our skin has twenty different meridians where the twelve regular meridians form the twelve skin zones. They act as a mirror to what's happening on the inside. Skin rashes, nodules, or lumps go through meridians into the inside of the organ system.

We need to look at the different locations of the skin issues to find out which organ system is affected, and look at the local appearance to ascertain a person's Yin or Yang type. Then we can make recommendation for how to address the issue with cooling or heating food. Once this is established, we look for the trigger (reaction) points to know where to apply acupressure or acupuncture.

The outside of the limbs and back of lower limbs is the Yang skin zone, which reflects issues of the small intestine and urinary bladder. The inside of the limbs and front of the trunk is the Yin skin zone, which reflects heart and kidney issues.

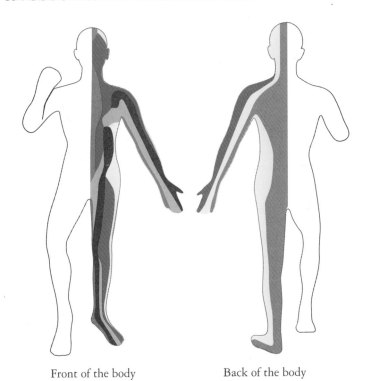

Front of the body   Back of the body

Color of Skin Zone	Sub-Category	Meridian	Treatment
	Taiyang	Bladder Meridian of Foot	Kidney system
		Small Intestine Meridian of Hand	Heart system
	Yangming	Large Intestine Meridian of Hand	Lung system
		Stomach Meridian of Foot	Spleen system
	Shaoyang	Gallbladder Meridian of Foot	Liver system
		Sanjiao Meridian of Hand	Heart system
	Taiyin	Lung Meridian of Hand	Lung system
		Spleen Meridian of Foot	Spleen system
	Shaoyin	Heart Meridian of Hand	Heart system
		Kidney Meridian of Foot	Kidney system
	Jueyin	Liver Meridian of Foot	Liver system
		Pericardium Meridian of Hand	Heart system

Skin zones and the related meridians.

If there is a red rash on the skin, then we ask if the patient feels itchy or sore or if there is a hot/burning sensation. The area outside the upper limb is the small intestine zone, as it is a hot rash

> **Example of trigger (reaction) points:**
> • Appendicitis: 2 cun (please refer to page 115 for more knowledge about cun) below the Zusanli point (ST 36), can treat early stage of appendicitis as opposed to having surgery.
> • Cholecystitis: 1 cun below the Yanglingquan point (GB 34), can limit infections as opposed to taking antibiotics.
> • Heart palpitations: ear heart point in the center of the ear to reduce the degree of pain and save time calling for help.

Academician Tang Zhaoyou has written a book about how both modern medicine and TCM work together. He notes, "I was a surgeon. I operated on a lot of patients. I didn't expect that several of my family members had a disease that needed surgery, but none of them were cured with surgery. In 1987, my 91-year-old mother had acute appendicitis perforation with diffuse peritonitis while I was abroad. My teacher came home to see my mother and suggested that she should operate immediately, but none of my family members agreed to the operation. By the time I got home, there was already a lot of fluid in my mother's abdominal cavity, but she was still determined not to be hospitalized. I could only give my mother an intravenous drip every day. I was supposed to use four bottles, but she only agreed to do one, and only one fourth of the normal dose of antibiotics was used in each bottle. I began to study the integration of traditional Chinese medicine and modern medicine in the late 1950s and participated in the publication of "116 Cases of Acute Appendicitis Treated with Acupuncture and Moxibustion" in the *Chinese Medical Journal* (*English Edition*). So, I used acupuncture twice a day to stimulate my mother's Zusanli point (ST 36). In this way, through the combination of traditional Chinese medicine and modern medicine, my mother's illness was cured in only 9 days. I also used acupuncture to treat my son and wife's appendicitis, and there was no recurrence." [1]

---

[1] Tang Zhaoyou: 《西学中，创中国新医学》, *Western Medicine Learning from Chinese Medicine, Creating New Chinese Medicine*, Shanghai Science and Technology Press, 2019.

and a Yang area, so we choose cooling foods, such as mung beans, watermelon, or honeysuckle. We can also use a cooling cream, such as cooling tiger balm and mint essential oils. For hot areas, TCM also uses skin needle therapy, applying the dermal needle of seven-star needles (*qi xing zhen*) method.

If there is some swelling or enlargement but the rash is the same color as the skin, this is an Yin type of issue. Itchiness may occur, but intermittently. We need food to regulate water metabolism and Warm/Hot food to speed up local circulation. We can also use a warming/heating cream, such as warm tiger balm and ginger essential oils.

2. Pulse Diagnosis

In TCM, feeling the pulse can give information about our digestive Qi, mental state, and kidney functions. For a "normal pulse," if there is enough digestive Qi, the strength level of the pulse will be in the middle and the width of the pulse will be medium. If there is good mental and spiritual energy, the pulse will be from 60 to 90 beats per minute with a regular rhythm. To indicate mental and kidney function, the pulse in the finger should be peaceful, flow smoothly and with power, and quite strong. For kidney function, we also check the third finger on the deepest level. If you can feel a smooth flow with power, this demonstrates strong kidney function.

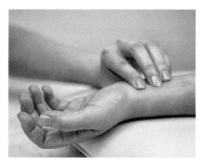

Feeling the pulse.

Left and right hand indicate different meridians and organs.

Left hand: *cun* (heart), *guan* (liver), *chi* (kidney Yin). Right hand: *cun* (lung), *guan* (spleen), *chi* (kidney Yang).

• Depth: Floating or Deep/Sinking

If you put light pressure over the radial artery, you will find the floating pulse. If you put medium pressure, you will find

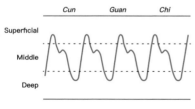

Normal pulse.

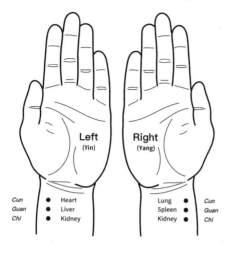

Basic pulse types: use index (*cun*), middle (*guan*), and ring (*chi*) fingers in the position of the styloid process area of the wrist.

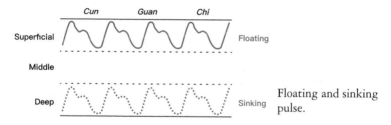

Floating and sinking pulse.

the middle pulse. With a more specific and strong pressure, you will find the deep pulse.

For illness that starts with external factors, we can understand its progression from the pulse depth. For example, at the onset of bronchitis, the pulse will likely be floating. Once this develops in the body, the depth of the pulse will be deeper. This indicates that the external factors have entered into the interior of the body.

For those illnesses that come from the internal organs, there may first be a deep pulse and early onset. This indicates that the issue started inside the body.

• Speed: Rapid or Slow

If it is above ninety beats per minute (Western medicine: heart murmur), this could be from infection, internal or inherited. A rapid pulse is an indicator of Heat or Fire, so we need to reduce the Heat and cool the body.

If the speed is less than sixty per minute, this is considered a

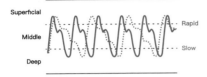

Rapid and slow pulse.

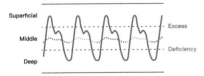

Excess and deficiency pulse.

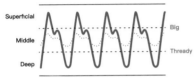

Big and thready pulse.

slow pulse (although this may be normal for athletes). For those who usually have a normal speed, if it slows to less than sixty, it indicates a Cold condition. If the body is exhausted or there is a blockage inside the heart, the pulse will slow down.

• Strength: Excess or Deficiency

If there is a strong pulse, the person has a good constitution. If there is less strength, it indicates a slightly weak body constitution. There is some variance between males and females, with males having a slightly stronger pulse. If the strength changes from normal to forceful, this is indicative of a hyper-excessive condition, usually caused by a foreign object invading the body, which we have to fight. If it becomes weaker and is below normal strength, it is a hypo-deficiency. There is usually a weakness of energy and Blood that will need strengthening and toning to improve the condition.

• Width: Big or Thready Pulse

A big pulse can be felt at all levels: superficial, middle, and deep. The opposite is a thready (or thin) pulse, which can only be felt on one level. If there is a big pulse, it is indicative of a Yang condition linked with Heat or excess syndromes. If there is a thready pulse, this usually indicates Yin conditions linked with Cold deficiency syndromes.

• Rhythm: Regular or Irregular

If the pulse is irregular and the speed is quick (above 90 per minute), the rhythm is hasty. This shows a Yang condition or excess syndrome, where the Hot factors are disturbing the heart, such as flu induced heart illness like myocarditis or heart-muscle infection. If the pulse is irregular and the speed is slow (below 60 per minute), it is considered a knotted pulse. This pulse is also an excess, but a Yin condition such as Blood stagnation, Cold, or Phlegm blockage.

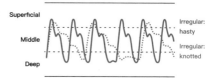

Irregular hasty pulse and irregular knotted pulse.

In clinical practice, these are often combined with an initial diagnosis. However, we can use this independently to understand any changes and identify early onset of illness prior to seeking medical advice.

Eight Principles of Differentiation

TCM notes there are a lot of exterior factors that can affect humans, even though most of the time we are not sick. Therefore, when we do become sick, it may be from something other than internal or external factors. Our body's healthy Qi also plays a role. If we work on our healthy Qi to make it balanced and active, we can stay healthy and not become ill. Being healthy depends on healthy Qi, as it can defend us from internal and external factors, until the factors of disease become too strong for our Qi to fight off.

The eight principles are interior and exterior, Cold and Hot, deficiency (empty) and excess (full), and Yin and Yang.

Clinical practise indicates that the eight principles are the theoretical basis for all identification of patterns and are applicable in every case, because they combines system body condition, symptoms, and signs and reflect on the pathogenesis of the illness. These principles are the foundation for all other methods of pattern formulation and the basic groundwork of pattern identification in TCM.

Identification of patterns according to the eight principles allow you to identify the location (interior and exterior), nature (Cold, Hot, pathologic conditions), characters (empty and full, healthy Qi being weak in morbid or deficiency, and factors in excess conditions), and categorization (Yin and Yang types), which later leads to the treatment principles and prognosis.

The Yin-Yang is the compendium of the rest of the eight principles. We use the eight principles to first identify the patterns when encountering an illness. The Yin and Yang syndromes can also be generalized as follows.

1. Yin and Yang

The Yin and Yang principle is used to generalize the categories. Yin is used to summarize interior, Cold, and deficiency. Yang is used to summarize exterior, Hot, and excess.

2. Interior and Exterior

Exterior conditions can be exterior Cold and exterior Hot. The onset of these illnesses is usually caused by external factors that appear in our body at the superficial level, such as skin, muscle, and surface rather than internal organs. Symptoms on the surface of the body indicate exterior Cold or exterior Hot conditions. Symptoms of exterior Cold present more chills than hot, a lack of sweat, a lack of thirst, a slow, superficial pulse, and no change in the tongue body and coating. Symptoms of exterior Hot present hot feelings or fever more than chills, sweat, thirst, rapid, superficial pulse, a normal or slightly red tongue body with yellow tongue coating.

Interior diseases can come from the exterior or start within the body, with chronic disease coming from inside of organ systems. Symptoms of interior Cold are feeling cold and a lack of warmth. This is then paired with the organ system. If it is stomach Cold, symptoms include a pale tongue with white coating, and the pulse will be slow and deep. Other symptoms include an intolerance for cold food and diarrhoea induced by eating cold things. Symptoms of interior Heat are feeling hot and fever, while not feeling cold. Accompanying this will be excessive perspiration, the need to drink cold beverages and eat cold or raw food, and constipation. The pulse will be rapid and deep, and the tongue body will be red or deep red with a thick yellow coating.

3. Cold and Hot

Cold syndromes mean that the nature of the disease is triggered by Cold factors and body constitution. If the outer appearance is pale or light color of the face, skin, and tongue body, this indicates Cold. The person usually has an aversion to cold and usually wants to drink warm or hot drinks and has an absence of thirst. Excretion from the five sense organs and nine openings (eyes, ears, mouth, nostrils, urethra, and anus) of the body are usually transparent, clear, and non-sticky and the volume is enlarged, such as loose stool, clear urine, frequent runny nose, tearing, and watery discharge. A slow pulse is a major indicator of Cold syndromes, except for athletes who are extremely fit and have a low resting heart rate. The tongue color is pale with white and a moist/watery coating.

Hot syndromes are redder in appearance, including red eyes, face, and complexion. Skin rashes are red in color and the tongue color is red. People with Hot syndromes often feel hot easily and often, are always thirsty with a preference for cold drinks, and all their excretions from different openings are more concentrated and yellow or green in color, such as yellow/green mucus from the sinuses, yellow discharge from the eyes or the ears, acne or pimples with yellow or bloody discharge, yellow or brown cough sputum, constipation, and deep yellow or scanty urine, and yellow vaginal discharge. A rapid pulse and red tongue body with yellow and dry coating are also symptoms.

4. Deficiency (Empty) and Excess (Full)

Excess syndrome is where the body has to fight in places where energy is blocked. This is shown by symptoms that are loud in volume, such as cough or vomiting, and a very strong pain. There is often distension or fullness in the chest and rib or abdominal area. The symptoms are usually sensitive to pressure. If you touch an area, the pain gets worse. Stool and urine are less frequent. The pulse is usually called an excess pulse. The tongue has a thick, sticky coating.

Deficiency syndromes show the opposite symptoms. The volume of coughing or vomiting is weak, there is a shortness of breath, a dislike of talking or speaking with a very low voice, a loss of interest, a poor memory, spontaneous or night sweats, insomnia or dream-disturbed sleep, menstruation two to three times per month or menstrual bleeding that cannot stop, dull aching such as headaches or chestaches, and responding well to pressure. Rest can improve this condition. The pulse is called deficiency pulse. The tongue has no coating or is very cracked, and the tongue is usually small or dry.

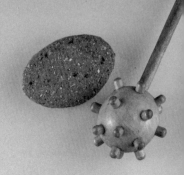

Part Two

TCM External Adjustment: The Mystery of Meridians and Acupoints

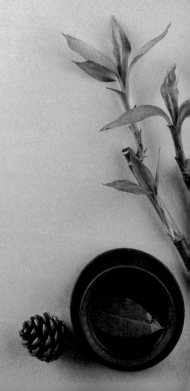

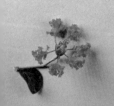

"We are what we connect."
—Chinese Prof. and PHD Dr. Wu Jianwei

The saying "You are what you eat and absorb" implies a one-sided relationship, indicating that the food and herbs we eat influence our body composition and health. In other words, something from outside affects the inside. Meridians, however, can go both ways. What we put into our bodies influences our outward appearance, while external manipulations on the body surface can influence the functioning of the internal organs. In order to ensure total health and harmony between the outside and inside, we need to use both external approaches (acupressure and acupuncture) and internal approaches (food and herbs). In this way we can regulate the entire system and achieve overall balance.

The meridian theory not only explains the phenomenon of the transmission of sensations along meridians that exists objectively in the human body, but also complements the internal organ, Qi, Blood, and Body Fluid theory to uniquely and profoundly explain people's physiological activities and pathological changes.

Using acupuncture anesthesia, mechanical stimulation, thermal stimulation (warm, hot), electrical stimulation, light stimulation, and magnetic stimulation through the meridians to achieve a significant improvement is becoming a daily application for prevention and treatment of ailments internationally.

Basic Questions (Su Wen) from *The Yellow Emperor's Internal Canon of Medicine* says, "The east is near the sea, and people there like to eat more fish and salty foods. Too much salty food will impair Blood, disturb water metabolism, and lead to illnesses such as carbuncles and ulcers, which can be cured by stone needle or stone scraping." It goes on to add, "The north has a longer winter, the landscape is more mountainous, and the climate is very cold. Moxibustion was created for use in this sort of environment." It further discusses the five common themes and indications, including stone needles (stone scraping), nine needles (acupuncture), moxibustion, Tuina (massage), and herbal medicine. Four of these are external forms of treatment, or non-medical therapy, while herbal medicine is a form of internal treatment, or medical therapy. These examples indicate that "various therapeutic methods are created from various environments and locations, along with people's constitutions." A wise doctor makes use of various methods and chooses the most suitable one. The reason different therapies can cure the same illness is that when doctors have fully understood the person's type and the disease changes, then the essential treatment is selected accordingly.

TCM is an external form of treatment that includes popular therapies such as acupuncture, moxibustion, Tuina, cupping, and Gua Sha scraping and topical applications of various types, all of which are based on an understanding of the meridian theory, or how to locate and stimulate reaction acupoints.

As you may have heard, TCM uses preventative treatment during the summer to regulate asthma, which attacks easily in the winter. The method of treatment begins with differentiating asthma types, then applying an appropriate topical herbal paste on the Feishu point (BL 13), Dazhui point (GV 14), and other points, repeating a few times. Similar methods can be used to prevent and treat arthritis or diarrhea. These methods have good results, reducing the severity of the illness or even curing it.

In this part, I will focus on:
• Acupuncture
• Moxibustion (warming method)
• Tuina (massage manipulation, as well as Chinese chiropractic practice)
• Cupping
• Gua Sha scraping
• Topical applications
All of these methods fall into the category of external adjustments.

Chapter Nine
How Are Meridians Related to Our Health

Since the 1970s, there has been a growth in international interest in the TCM meridian theory and related treatments. Much research has been conducted, offering compelling evidence that acupuncture can be used to control certain types of pain, regulate the immune system to control inflammation, and improve and balance the internal organs. As such, it has gained popularity and is now in widespread use across the world.

In TCM, acupuncture and moxibustion are as important as the primary methods of food therapy and herbal remedies. In the Ming dynasty (1368–1644), a well-known doctor said, "If you don't study or understand the twelve regular meridians, when you practice or talk about diagnosis and treatment, you may easily make mistakes." For this reason, TCM doctors place strong emphasis on food, herbs, meridian theory, and methods such as acupuncture, Tuina, moxibustion, Gua Sha scraping, and cupping, all of which are related. In international medicine, these methods are now accepted and understood, and are now implemented more broadly, especially using food and Tuina to address health issues, since changes in diet and generation of energy flow are relatively easy to achieve.

Foundational TCM books such as *The Yellow Emperors' Internal Canon of Medicine* note that meridian-related therapies can treat all types of disease. They can regulate conditions of excess and weakness (hypo and hyper) and can provide essential information for future prognosis.

To understand the concept of meridians, we need to understand the complex network between the meridians and internal organs. Much like a city, there are multiple connections and ways for effective functioning. Using this analogy, cities are our organs and the transportation infrastructure (roads, highways, waterways, and air

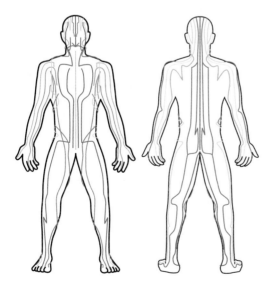

Main meridians on the body. Front (left) and back (right).

paths) are meridians. This comprehensive network makes up a city that functions on all levels. It is three dimensional and exists at multiple levels, not just on a flat plane. Similarly, the meridian system connects all parts of the body and creates pathways for information and energy to flow so that the body may operate effectively and keep healthy.

When we have a health issue, we must first identify whether it is acute or chronic. If it is acute and severe, we may be able to diagnose it immediately and follow treatment principles immediately, using an antidote against the disease as food and acupuncture therapies are applied. If the issue is chronic and recurring, we may immediately adjust past medical treatments, adding meridian therapy and changing the diet to include more balanced and nutritional foods. If there are skin or joint issues, topical use of plant soaks or herbal baths can be applied. These methods can help open meridian blockages and relieve symptoms.

The relationship between the meridians and human health shows up in three areas: prevention methods, diagnosis, and treatment.

Healthcare and Prevention Methods

Meridian natural therapy can be used in many ways, a few of which will be described here, with a focus on the use of meridian therapy to improve health.

1. Healthcare and Prevention Methods Based on Previous Medical Experience and Weaknesses

From our own previous experiences of being ill, we know where our weaknesses are in the body. For example, when contracting a cold or flu, it may affect the nose and sinuses in one patient, but affect the stomach and appetite in another.

If Cold always affects the nose and sinuses, the Lung Meridian needs strengthening. If this does not happen frequently, it is considered normal, but when it happens up to 4 to 5 times a year or occurs continuously without breaks, it must be addressed. To strengthen lungs and prevent illness, we can eat almonds, pears, lotus roots, or lotus seeds. We can also touch or massage meridian points such as the Chize point (LU 5) and Lieque point (LU 7). Another method for treating such ailments is breathing exercises, which can also strengthen the lungs by building lung capacity.

If Cold or stress always affects the stomach, causing symptoms such as stomachache, bloating, and diarrhea, the stomach and spleen system needs strengthening. To do so, we can eat ginger, whole grains such as glutinous rice, buckwheat, congee, or oats, root vegetables such as yams, or beans like lentils. We can also treat the meridians through application of moxa on the Zusanli point (ST 36) and localized massage around the stomach or belly button. Muscle exercises such as stretching can also strengthen the digestive system.

2. Healthcare and Preventive Methods Based on Genetic and Inherited Conditions (Family History)

If we know what conditions have been experienced by previous generations in one's family, we can take measures to prevent the same conditions occurring in the patient's life. Family history is a good indicator of potential health issues, so we should look to our parents and grandparents (or even immediate relatives) to identify potential weak areas.

A history of high cholesterol would indicate the need to strengthen the liver system. To strengthen the liver, massage from the underarm towards the hip, following the rib line to the belly button. Practice deep breathing exercises for 10 to 15 minutes, twice a day. Alternatively, massage from the temple, following the Gallbladder Meridian, and the Fengchi (GB 20) and Jianjing points (GB 21) to the back of the head to relax the liver. This method will address symptoms

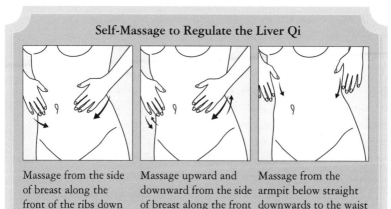

Self-Massage to Regulate the Liver Qi

Massage from the side of breast along the front of the ribs down following the natural curves, repeat 20 times.

Massage upward and downward from the side of breast along the front of the ribs down to the belly, repeat 20 times.

Massage from the armpit below straight downwards to the waist bone, repeat 20 times.

such as migraines, sore eyes, and red eyes. To strengthen the liver, one can eat asparagus, alfalfa sprouts, and artichokes.

If there is a history of joint problems, such as the hip or toe joints, or the development of osteoporosis (during menopause), we must tone the kidney system.

Some preventative methods for joint problems include delaying menopause by toning the kidneys and related organ system with food (starting from the age of around 42 or 45). For example, one can eat more nuts and seeds in winter, and eat more black beans and spinach after each menstrual cycle. One must also ensure that calcium levels and vitamin D are normal and avoid over-exercise, as this also uses kidney Essence. Note that the level of exercise is highly dependent on the individual baseline level, age range, and season. For example, some people are more suited to running a half marathon than a full marathon, or one hour of strength training rather than two hours of strength training.

Many meridian points for the kidney are in the feet. Thus, foot reflexology can be an effective method to strengthen the kidney. To address these problems, one can massage the Yongquan point (KI 1) with essential oils, which will also help with insomnia and disturbed sleep.

Diagnosis According to the Meridian Points and Distribution Area of the Meridians

In TCM, we use the meridians to diagnose and identify certain syndromes. There are many points on the surface of the body that are useful for understanding what is happening inside the body.

Meridians and points are also the reactor points of human physiology and pathology. The part of the meridian points on the surface of body is called *shu xue*. When you use acupuncture, moxibustion, massage, cupping, scraping, and other methods to stimulate the body's surface points, it will affect the whole meridian or a few of the meridian's energy and blood movements, while also influencing the inner organs.

At the same time, internal changes will be reflected through the channels and collaterals to the body surface of the involved meridians or at certain points. For instance, markers like rashes, acne, or pigmentation on the side of one's face are connected with the Stomach Meridian. Nodules on the side of the neck indicate gallbladder Heat and high stress periods. It also shows tenderness and develops muscle strains and lumps, indicating pathogenic changes within the body system. When there is an onset of cholecystitis or gallstone's disease, the Dannang point (EX-LE 6, one cun below the Yanglingquan point, GB 34) has a reaction point to be diagnosed and where one may apply treatment. The early stages of appendicitis start from a migration of abnormal pain. There is severe pain with the sudden release of deep pressure to the right lower abdomen (rebound tenderness). At the same time, the right leg cannot be stretched to full length and the Lanwei point (EX-LE 7, 2 cun below the Zusanli point, ST 36) will have a reaction point. Therefore, we should regularly check the surface of our skin around these major points to see if there is any change.

Many types of pain are triggered by sports, incorrect posture, or improper movements. Modern English calls these "trigger points," as we understand the reaction points, or "Ashi points." Meridian related treatments to those points can have a wonderful effect.

A large amount of clinical data proves that each acupoint has a certain specificity. Using acupuncture points that are positive for pathological reactions and applying acupuncture treatments to certain disease often achieve very satisfactory results.

For example, gastric diseases often have pathological reactions at two acupoints, the Weishu point (BL 21) and the Liangqiu point (ST 34). A fatty liver has pathological reactions with the Ganshu point (BL 18) and the Qimen point (LR 14) on the Liver Meridian. Using these points for acupuncture treatment, the effect of the treatment is obvious and relatively rapid.

Distribution areas of the meridians can also help in diagnosis. For example, if you have a headache, we first look at the relevant meridians. If the headache occurs in the forehead, it is the Yangming Meridian, which is linked to the stomach or large intestine. If the headache is at the back of the head, it is the Taiyang Meridian of the Urinary Bladder. And if at the side, it is the Shaoyang Meridian of the Gallbladder or *Sanjiao*. Once we know the related meridians and organs, we can then diagnose and apply the right treatment.

Meridians are also a way for external stimuli (bacteria/virus/weather) to attack internal organs from the surface. These factors come into the body through our skin, muscles and meridians. Once we

Body Length Measurement

An important means of locating acupoints is through "body length" measurements. This system is an ingenious way by which anyone can measure and locate acupoints on his or her own body. Since everyone's body is of different size and shape, using a measurement system specific to the individual makes finding the points easy.

The process starts with the measurement of one cun. This is done in two ways:

• Using the width of the distal inter-phalangeal joint of the thumb.

• Using the distance between the distal and proximal interphalangeal joints of the third (middle) finger.

All other specific measurements are outlined in the diagrams below. If in doubt when measuring, the thumb (1 cun) or the four-finger method (3 cun) may be used alternatively.

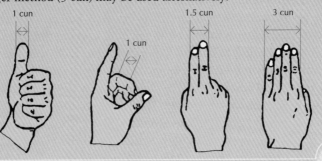

know which meridian has been attacked, we can address the relevant area and understand what is happening in the body. Dr. Zhang Zhongjing of Eastern Han dynasty in his book *Treatise on Cold Damage* (*Shang Han Lun*) notes that for an acute flu, the Taiyang Meridian pattern is at the exterior level, the Shaoyang Meridian pattern is in between the exterior and the interior, and the Yangming Meridian pattern is at the interior level. Based on this understanding, the treatment principles and methods are different for each case.

For eczema, rheumatoid arthritis, and diabetes, a change happens inside first, then surfaces on the outside. Diabetes primarily starts from the dysfunction of an organ, such as the pancreas, but can further affect other organs if not addressed properly, moving to the kidney or the heart, then causing muscle and nerve damage on the legs and toes.

Meridian-Based Treatment

The meridians are also functional units of the exchange of energy and Blood. This refers to the regulation of energy and Blood in the meridians, which can affect the function of the viscera. It provides two-way adjustment between each internal organ. Therefore, the five organ system was formed and functions. The biological link of the whole can help the body maintain a state of internal and external stability and balance. By applying meridian-related therapies, we can further balance up and down, left and right, outer and inner, and Yin and Yang in the body. There are many forms of meridian treatment, including acupuncture, ear acupuncture, moxibustion, massage, cupping, Gua Sha scraping, and Qigong. They are all based on the meridian theory and its application (see more details about these applications in the following chapters).

Food and herbal treatments can target the meridians, and then enter the organs. Therefore, when you have hives, you should note whether they are located on the Yin or Yang side of limbs. When applying food and herbal therapy, you must choose according to the organs and related meridians. If the hives are on the Lung Meridian, it indicates Dryness in the lungs, for which lily bulbs or almonds are the best foods. If the hives are on the outer leg, it indicates Heat in the Stomach or Gallbladder Meridian, and dandelion or sweet wormwood (*qing hao*) are recommended. If you have a tendency to feel cold in the stomach area, it is recommended to add ginger tea to your diet. You may also add ginger and spring onion to food. To maximize the benefits, use these ingredients for at least one month. Many foods enter both organs and meridians. For instance, peppers affect the Stomach Meridian and the stomach, while sunflower seeds affect the Spleen Meridian and

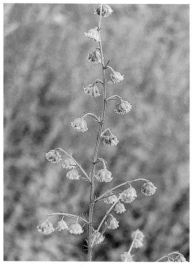

Sweet wormwood.

the spleen. Kidney beans, naturally, affect the Kidney Meridian and the kidney, and coffee affects the heart and its meridian.

There is a close relationship between foods, herbs, and meridians which is called "Channels of Entry." This refers to the selective effect of plants on a certain part of the body. Mainly, it has a significant effect on a certain meridian (the viscera and its meridian) or a few meridians, while it has less or no effect on other meridians. Like cooling herbs, although they all have Heat-clearing effects, their range of action is either partial to clearing the lung or clearing the heart, each of which has its own advantages. It is the same with the tonic. There are differences such as toning the lungs, toning the spleen, and toning the kidneys. Therefore, the therapeutic effects of various herbs on various parts of the body are further summarized and systemized, which forms the theory of Channels of Entry (*gui jing*). For example, if we have a headache in a certain place, as described above (forehead, side of head, back of head), we can find food and herbal remedies to target the specific meridians. For treating migraines, we can drink tea made of 3 grams of chrysanthemum and 5 grams of mulberry leaves.

If we understand the meridian theory, we can then take action before the disease develops, ensuring our stable happiness and health.

A TCM doctor will prescribe certain foods according to the relevant meridian and diagnosis. Basil is an example of an herb that has a variety of functions to address health issues. In TCM, basil is a Warm, Pungent herb. It enters the Lung, Spleen, and Stomach Meridians and goes to the lung, spleen, and stomach organs.

The first function and application of this herb is to expel Wind and move the energy of the meridian and organ, so this can treat common colds with headaches, fever, cough, chest pressure, and even summer colds. For summer colds, we can use 6 grams of basil and 3 grams of raw licorice to make tea or for cooking. For common colds with a headache centered on the forehead, we can use 6 grams basil and add 2 grams fresh perilla leaves to

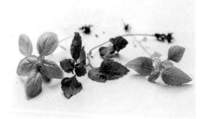
Basil has a variety of functions.

make a tea or for cooking.

The second function of this herb is to remove Dampness and harmonize the digestive function. It can be used to aid the appetite by adding basil to cooking or making tea. It can also help people with toothaches and bad breath. Just put few fresh leaves in the mouth. In addition, it is used to help stomach and abdominal bloating, nausea, and loose stool. Combine 10 to 12 grams of basil with 4 to 6 grams of ginger (dried). To address nausea, add 2 teaspoons of fresh sugarcane juice (or maple syrup), 1 teaspoons of fresh basil (bitter and sweet together), and drink them together.

The third application is for detoxification. To remove toxins, basil can be used as a topical application. For example, if a baby has eczema or a rash from insects, basil can be used topically to remove the toxin. For dandruff, mix together basil and vinegar and apply to the head.

In summary, the meridian theory is very important for our health. Whether it is in the prevention, diagnosis, or treatment of diseases, it plays a unique and comprehensive role, among which prevention is always better than cure.

Chapter Ten
Meridian Maps and Self-Adjustment Points

The meridians form the material structure of the human body. In organizational structure, the meridian system consists of the large trunk, small branch, and the internal and external inter-connection parts of the meridians.

The large trunk consists mainly of 12 regular meridians and eight extraordinary vessels. The small branch mainly consists of 15 small collaterals. This book introduces the main meridians.

The internal organs are interconnected with the external limbs, joints, muscles, ligaments, and skin of the entire body through the meridians. The perspective of TCM will lead you into the realm of the human body. Our organ system is similar to the engine of a car. The nutrients in our bodies, such as Qi, Blood, Body Fluid, and Essence, are like the oil in a car. The meridian system in our body can be likened to automotive circuits, tubing, and all of the connecting parts, such as the accelerator, brakes, air conditioning, and so on. They all must have interconnected parts to link them as a whole, just as the entire cell, tissues of the human body, limbs, and skin, need the meridians to connect them.

The meridians are energy networks functioning as a transportation system, carrying information to and from each organ. The meridians transport Qi, Blood, Body Fluids, Essence and nutrition to every part of the body. They communicate with the upper and lower surfaces and connect the sense organs, tissue, and viscera. There are twelve paired meridians, relating to the *zang* and *fu* organs, as well as two single vessels, relating to the Governing Vessel and the Conception Vessel, the main rivers of the body's Yin and Yang energies (plus six other extraordinary vessels).

According to the theoretical framework of TCM, the external belongs to the Yang, which in conjunction with the Yin is the balancing force in nature. In general, Yang is associated with the male, activity and Heat. The external can be subdivided into the three Yang meridian channels, the Yangming, the Shaoyang, and the Taiyang. Yang meridians are found mostly on the back of the hands, the outside of the arms and legs, and the back of the trunk (one exception is Stomach Meridian which distributes on the front of the trunk). They can influence our *fu* organs. The internal belongs to the Yin, which is traditionally associated with the female, dark, and the Cold. It can be further divided into the three Yin meridian channels, the Taiyin, the Jueyin, and the Shaoyin. The Yin meridians are distributed on the palm side of the hands, the inside of the arms and legs, and the front of the trunk. They can influence our *zang* organs. In application, for example, if there is an exterior manifestation, such as eczema on the face, we will conduct treatment on the Yang meridian points, as they travel to the face.

One way to understand the relationship between the inside and outside of the body is to think about the effect of a massage. After a massage, most people not only feel relaxed in the skin or outer muscles, but also have an overall sense of well-being. Manipulating the body's surface energy level is beneficial to the inside of the body as well.

There are many other examples of this linkage, including the practice of holding premature babies to strengthen their immune systems and of energy-healing techniques such as Qigong massage and Reiki. Reiki is a type of therapy in which the practitioner uses his

Category of Meridians			
Category	Sub-Category	Meridian	Yin-Yang Paired Meridian
Yang	Yangming	Large Intestine Meridian of the Hand	Lung Meridian of the Hand
		Stomach Meridian of the Foot	Spleen Meridian of the Foot
	Shaoyang	Gallbladder Meridian of the Foot	Liver Meridian of the Foot
		Sanjiao Meridian of the Hand	Pericardium Meridian of the Hand
	Taiyang	Bladder Meridian of the Foot	Kidney Meridian of the Foot
		Small Intestine Meridian of the Hand	Heart Meridian of the Hand
Yin	Taiyin	Lung Meridian of the Hand	Large Intestine Meridian of the Hand
		Spleen Meridian of the Foot	Stomach Meridian of the Foot
	Jueyin	Liver Meridian of the Foot	Gallbladder Meridian of the Foot
		Pericardium Meridian of the Hand	*Sanjiao* Meridian of the Hand
	Shaoyin	Heart Meridian of the Hand	Small Intestine Meridian of the Hand
		Kidney Meridian of the Foot	Bladder Meridian of the Foot

Category of meridians.

or her own energy to alter the patient's energy. This occurs without touching the patient and is similar to Qigong therapy. Intimate touch between lovers, or even just hugging (one study has shown that hugs increase levels of oxytocin and reduce blood pressure), is another example of how surface contact can provide multiple levels of healing deep within the body.

The direction, cross area, and distribution of twelve regular meridians is as follows (also refer to the diagram on the left):

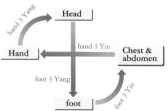

Direction of meridians.

Hand 3 Yin, from chest to hand.

Hand 3 Yang, from hand to head.

Foot 3 Yang, from head to foot.

Foot 3 Yin, from foot to abdomen.

Meridian Maps

Having acquired some basic knowledge of the fourteen meridians and collaterals, along with the direction and distribution of the Yin and Yang meridians, you can carry out self-adjustment through massage and tapping of certain meridians to treat some symptoms and discomfort (which are listed below, corresponding to each meridian). The general approach is to press the meridian to discover its sensitive points, then massage or tap it, or press or tap wherever you feel discomfort or along that meridian. Please be noted that all recommended acupoints for health care in this book can be found in these meridian maps for their location.

1. Yangming Large Intestine Meridian of the Hand (LI)

Examples of the main treatment of syndromes include constipation, pain along the meridian lines (on elbow), and stiffness in the neck and shoulders.

2. Taiyin Lung Meridian of the Hand (LU)

Examples of main treatment of syndromes include nasal sinusitis, sore throat, cough, and asthmatic breathing.

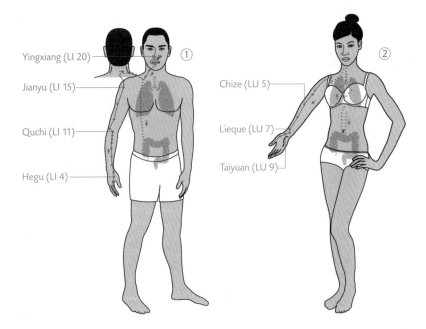

Yingxiang (LI 20)
Jianyu (LI 15)
Quchi (LI 11)
Hegu (LI 4)
①

Chize (LU 5)
Lieque (LU 7)
Taiyuan (LU 9)
②

3. Shaoyang *Sanjiao* (Triple Energizer) Meridian of the Hand (TE)

Examples of the main treatment of syndromes include pain, numbness, and swelling along the meridian lines, migraine, and tinnitus.

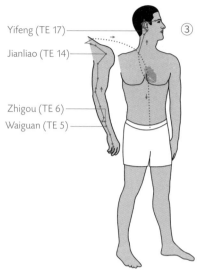

Yifeng (TE 17)

Jianliao (TE 14)

Zhigou (TE 6)

Waiguan (TE 5)

③

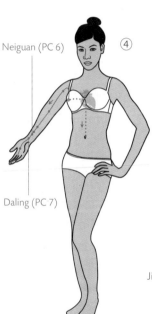

Neiguan (PC 6)

④

Daling (PC 7)

4. Jueyin Pericardium Meridian of the Hand (PC)

Examples of the main treatment of syndromes include palpitation and anxiety, chest pressure, sickness, and vomiting.

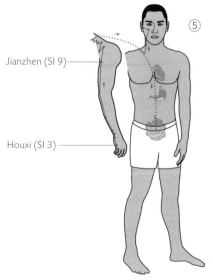

Jianzhen (SI 9)

Houxi (SI 3)

⑤

5. Taiyang Small Intestine Meridian of the Hand (SI)

Examples of the main treatment of syndromes include acute sprain of the neck and upper back, shoulder and soft tissue aches and stiffness, and insufficient lactation.

6. Shaoyin Heart Meridian of the Hand (HT)

Examples of the main treatment of syndromes include restlessness and insomnia, mouth and tongue ulcers, poor memory, and depression.

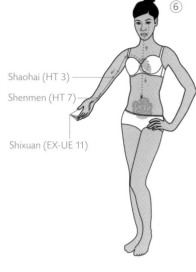

Shaohai (HT 3)

Shenmen (HT 7)

Shixuan (EX-UE 11)

Taiyang (EX-HN 5)

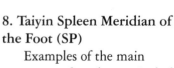

Sibai (ST 2)

Tianshu (ST 25)

Liangqiu (ST 34)
Dubi (ST 35)
Zusanli (ST 36)

Lanwei (EX-LE 7)

7. Yangming Stomach Meridian of the Foot (ST)

Examples of the main treatment of syndromes include facial wrinkles, head, tooth, or abdominal pain and swelling, and appendicitis.

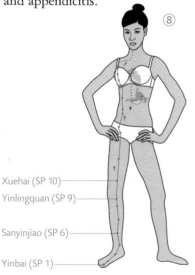

8. Taiyin Spleen Meridian of the Foot (SP)

Examples of the main treatment of syndromes include abdominal bloating, soft stool, edema and itching, and irregular menstruation.

Xuehai (SP 10)

Yinlingquan (SP 9)

Sanyinjiao (SP 6)

Yinbai (SP 1)

9. Shaoyang Gallbladder Meridian of the Foot (GB)

Examples of the main treatment of syndromes include migraine, sore eyes, bitter taste in the mouth, jaundice, tendon and joints issues along the meridian lines.

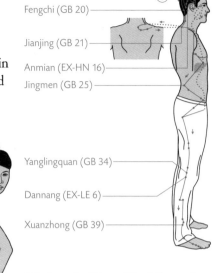

Fengchi (GB 20)
Jianjing (GB 21)
Anmian (EX-HN 16)
Jingmen (GB 25)
Yanglingquan (GB 34)
Dannang (EX-LE 6)
Xuanzhong (GB 39)

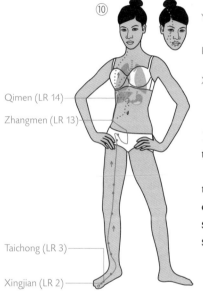

Qimen (LR 14)
Zhangmen (LR 13)
Taichong (LR 3)
Xingjian (LR 2)

10. Jueyin Liver Meridian of the Foot (LR)

Examples of the main treatment of syndromes include dizziness and blurred vision, sore breasts and painful periods, spasms and shivers (trembling).

11. Taiyang Bladder Meridian of the Foot (BL)

Examples of the main treatment of syndromes include sore eyes, organ conditions, and muscle, tendon, and joint issues along the meridian lines.

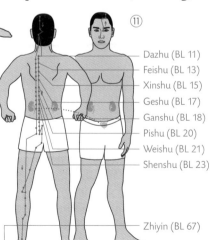

Dazhu (BL 11)
Feishu (BL 13)
Xinshu (BL 15)
Geshu (BL 17)
Ganshu (BL 18)
Pishu (BL 20)
Weishu (BL 21)
Shenshu (BL 23)
Zhiyin (BL 67)

12. Shaoyin Kidney Meridian of the Foot (KI)

Examples of the main treatment of syndromes include back, leg, and knee weakness, muscle softness, hot flashes and sweating, and frequent urine.

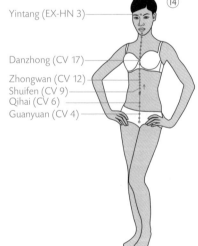

Taixi (KI 3)

Yongquan (KI 1)

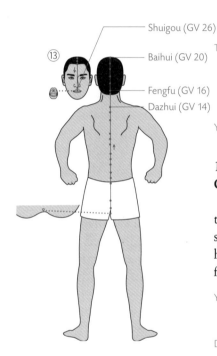

Shuigou (GV 26)
Baihui (GV 20)
Fengfu (GV 16)
Dazhui (GV 14)

13. The Extraordinary Vessel: Governing Vessel (GV)

Examples of the main treatment of syndromes include stiffness and aching of the spine, hemorrhoids, headaches and fainting.

Yintang (EX-HN 3)

Danzhong (CV 17)
Zhongwan (CV 12)
Shuifen (CV 9)
Qihai (CV 6)
Guanyuan (CV 4)

14. The Extraordinary Vessel: Conception Vessel (CV)

Examples of the main treatment of syndromes include asthma, stomach pain, infertility, and low libido.

Meridian Acupoints

Acupoints are specific locations on the body surface where an acupuncture needle is inserted or pressure is applied for therapeutic purposes. Many of those points can be connected to a meridian. The viscera, meridians, and acupoints in the interior and exterior form

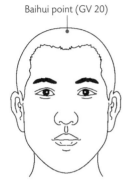

Baihui point.

an organic whole, with a close relation and harmonious unity.

Acupoints have three main functions. The first is a proximal curative effect or local action. This is the common characteristic that all acupuncture points have. That is to say, all acupoints can treat diseases of the local and adjacent tissues and organs, especially the acupoints located on the head, face, and trunk. For instance, the Baihui point (GV 20) located on the head can treat headaches and vertigo.

The second is a distal curative effect. This is the feature of the fourteen meridian points, especially the points of the twelve meridians located below the elbows and knees. These points can treat regional illnesses as well as the disorders of the internal organs and tissues associated with the meridians along their distribution. Some can treat discomfort throughout the body. For example, the Zusanli point (ST 36), located on the shank, can treat leg and knee pain and can help with stomachaches and lightheadedness. It is also a key point for cultivating health to reinforce the body's resistance.

The third is a two-way curative effect. This indicates that some of the points have adapted to the original condition. For instance, work on the Neiguan point (PC 6) can reduce the heartbeat if it is too fast or increase the heart rate if it is too slow.

Helpful Self-Adjustment Acupressure Points

Work on the meridian points affects the function of the internal organs through the movement of Qi and Blood in the corresponding meridians. Each acupoint plays a specific role in the treatment of diseases.

The surface acupoints on meridians can be roughly divided into three categories: The first meridian points are those located on the twelve meridians and the governing and conception vessels. These points are the main part in the acupoint family and are the most frequently used points.

The second are extraordinary points, referring to the points not included in those belonging to the fourteen meridians. They have definite locations and names and are effective in treating certain illnesses. For example, the Anmian point (EX-HN 16) has strong sleep-regulating function.

The third are Ashi points, or tender spots, painful points, sensitive spots, or reaction points. Some doctors call these "trigger points." Such points have no fixed location, no pertaining meridians, and no name.

Some self-adjustment acupressure points that can help you address discomfort or ailments in daily life are included below. You can find their locations on the meridian maps in the previous section Please be noted that all the points are symmetrical on the body, but they are only presented on one side in these maps.

• Shixuan (Diffusing Point 十宣 , EX-UE 11): on the tips of the ten fingers, a few millimeters from the nail.

Indications: revive unconscious patients, treat those in shock, or have fainted, suffering from a seizure, or are in a coma.

• Yintang (Seal Hall 印堂 , GV 29): between the eyebrows, equidistant between them.

Indications: muddled head, headache, insomnia, and infantile convulsions. May be used to calm the mind and allay anxiety.

• Shuigou (Water Trough 水沟 , GV 26): above the upper lip, in the crease, one third of the distance from the base of the nasal septum to the center of the red skin on the upper lip.

Indications: mental disorders, epilepsy, hysteria, infantile convulsions, coma, and stroke.

• Daling (Big Mound 大陵 , PC 7): between two tendons at the midpoint of the wrist and palm transverse crease.

Indications: heart pain, palpitations, mental disorders, epilepsy, stuffy chest, pain in the rib region, insomnia, irritability, and stomachaches.

• Hegu (Union Valley 合谷 , LI 4): on the fleshy part of the hand between the thumb and forefinger. Using your left hand, match the first crease of the thumb joint to the edge of the middle fleshy portion of the right hand and pressing down on the thumb. Meet the forefinger of the left hand on the opposite side and press.

Indications: ache points, headaches, muddled head, swelling of the face, and sore throat. Can be used to open the chest for stagnated lung Qi to harmonize with the large intestine, and for menstrual blockage.

• Shenmen (Spirit Gate 神门 , HT 7): between the first and second line of the wrist in the depression at the upper forearm to the small finger side of the hand, inside the wrist crease of the large tendon.

Indications: heart pain, irritability, palpitations, insomnia, epilepsy. Can also aid in balancing the heart and liver.

• Fengchi (Wind Pool 风池 , GB 20): on the posterior aspect of the neck, below the occipital bone, on the hairline in a depression on the outer area of the largest tendon.

Indications: headache along the Shaoyang Meridian or from the back area, vertigo, difficulty sleeping, blurred vision, tinnitus, convulsions, epilepsy, nasal blockage, painful stiffness of the neck.

• Baihui (Hundred Convergences 百会 , GV 20): on the middle line of the head, at the cross section of the line running from the nose to the base of the head and both ears, at the top of the head.

Indications: headache along the Jueyin Meridian, mental disorders, prolapse of the internal organs, coma, vertigo.

• Anmian (Quiet Sleep 安眠 , EX-HN 16): at the middle point of the depression behind the ear next to the ear lobe and the Fengchi point (GB 20).

Indications: insomnia, irritability, migraine, palpitations, mental disorder, light and disturbed sleep.

• Shaohai (Lesser Sea 少海 , HT 3): at the bend of the elbow, at the medial end of the cubital crease, in the depression just anterior to the medial epicondyle of the humerus.

Indications: heart pain, numbness of the arm, tremors in the hand, armpit and rib pain.

• Xingjian (Moving Between 行间 , LR 2): on the dorsal aspect of the foot, on the web area between the first and second toe at the line coloration of white and pink skin.

Indications: irregular menstruation, insomnia, epilepsy, convulsions, premenstrual tension, swelling and painful chest, distension of the abdominals, pain and fullness of the rib area, swelling and pain of the eyes, dizziness, and vertigo.

• Yongquan (Spring Water 涌泉 , KI 1): on the middle front deeper sole, at the junction of the anterior one third and posterior two thirds of the sole.

Indications: dizziness and headache, loss of voice and dryness of the tongue, fever, and loss of consciousness.

• Guanyuan (Gate of Original Qi 关元 , CV 4): on the midline of the abdomen, 3 cun below the umbilicus.

Indications: frequent urination or retention of urine, irregular menstruation, uterine bleeding, indigestion, diarrhea.

• Jianzhen (Upright Shoulder 肩贞 , SI 9): on the posterior aspect of the upper arm, 1 cun directly above the back of the armpit fold.

Indications: shoulder blade pain, arm unable to be raised, arm numbness and pain, tinnitus, and deafness.

• Sibai (Four Whites 四白 , ST 2): in the depression of the orifice under the eye socket, under the central line of the eyeball.

Indications: eye wrinkle and eye bag, red, sore and swollen eyes, facial paralysis.

• Yingxiang (Welcoming Perfume 迎香 , LI 20): 0.5 cun beside the wing of nose, in the nasolabial groove.

Indications: hay fever, itchiness and swelling, nasal obstruction.

• Lieque (Broken Sequence 列缺 , LU 7): 1.5 cun proximal to the wrist, in a crevice on the lateral edge of the radius just proximal to the styloid process.

Indications: hay fever, sore throat, clenched jaws, productive cough and asthma, headache and stiff neck, deviated eyes and mouth.

• Taichong (Supreme Surge 太冲 , LR 3): on the dorsal aspect of the foot, in the depression distal to the junction of the first and second metatarsal bones.

Indications: headache, swelling and pain of eyes, insomnia, rib-side distention.

• Zusanli (Leg Three Li 足三里 , ST 36): on the anterior aspect of the lower leg, 3 cun inferior to Dubi (ST 35), about one finger width lateral to the tibia.

Indications: stomach pain, indigestion, diarrhea, dizziness and aversion to cold, cold legs.

• Sanyinjiao (Three Yin Intersection 三阴交 , SP 6): on the rear edge of the shin bone, 3 cun above the ankle.

Indications: abdominal distention, diarrhea, uterine bleeding, menstrual irregularities, insomnia, and infertility.

• Taixi (Great Ravine 太溪 , KI 3): at the ankle joint, midway between the tip of the inside ankle and tendon.

Indications: sore throat, toothache, dizziness, aging, palpitation, waking up earlier than usual, menstrual irregularities, coughing up blood, asthma, and pain in the lower back.

• Shenshu (Kidney Transport 肾俞 , BL 23): on the lower back, level with the inferior border of the spine process of the two lumbar vertebra, 1.5 cun lateral of the midline.

Indications: seminal emission, menstrual irregularities, vaginal discharge, lumbar pain, tinnitus, short breath, and diarrhea.

• Neiguan (Inner Gate 内关 , PC 6): between two tendons, 2 cun over the wrist transverse crease.

Indications: stomach bloating, chest pain, palpitation, and mania.

• Tianshu (Celestial Pivot 天枢 , ST 25): on the abdomen, level with the center of the umbilicus, 2 cun lateral to the midline.

Indications: abdominal pain, constipation, weight gain, water swelling, and menstrual irregularities.

• Zhigou (Branch Ditch 支沟 , SJ 6): on the palmar side of the forearm, 3 cun proximal above the wrist, midway between the two bones.

Indications: abdominal pain and constipation, sudden loss of voice, oppressive glooms in the chest and stomach duct, and rib-side pain.

• Xuehai (Sea of Blood 血海 , SP 10): (1) When the knee is flexed, the point is 2 cun above the medial superior border of the patella on the bulge of the medial portion of quadriceps femoris. (2) When the knee is flexed, cup your right palm to the patient's left knee, with the thumb on the medial side and other 4 fingers directed proximally and the thumb forming an angle of 45 degrees with the index finger. The point is where the tip of your thumb rests.

Indications: eczema, rash, uterine bleeding, pain in the thigh, itching skin, and irregular menstruation.

• Houxi (Back Ravine 后溪 , SI 3): on the little finger side of the palmar, proximal to the head of the fifth bone, at the border of the red & white flesh.

Indications: headache, stiff neck, epilepsy, night sweating, and back pain.

• Waiguan (Outer Pass 外关 , SJ 5): on the palmar side of the forearm, 2 cun proximal above the wrist, midway between the two bones.

Indications: heat disease, headache and stiff neck, tinnitus, pain of the meridian line area, and tremors in the hand.

Eight Confluent Points

These are eight confluent points, located on the trunk and four limbs below the elbows and the knees. These are the areas where the Essence, Qi of *zang* organs, *fu* organs, Qi, Blood, tendons, vessels, bones, and marrow converge.

The eight confluent points can be used as preferential acupoints to treat eight categories of diseases, such as viscera, Qi, Blood, tendons, bones, vessels, and marrow disorder, and for treating illness of the meridian where they locate.

• Zhongwan (Middle Stomach 中脘 , CV 12, or gathering Yang organs): on the upper abdomen, on the middle line, two fingers below the chest bone, in the depression.

Indications: stomachache, abdominal distension, nausea, vomiting, acid regurgitation, diarrhea, jaundice, and indigestion caused by stress.

• Zhangmen (Chapter Gate 章门 , LR 13, or gathering Yin organs): on the lateral aspect of the abdomen, approximately on the midaxillary line, immediately below the tip of the eleventh rib.

Indications: loose stool and abdominal distension, retention of food, belching, and fullness in the epigastrium. It is the main point for harmonizing the liver and spleen.

• Xuanzhong (Hanging Bell 悬钟 , GB 39, or gathering marrow): 3 cun above the tip of outside ankle.

Indications: stiffness and pain in the neck, ribs, knee, and thigh, and distention or fullness of chest and abdomen.

• Yanglingquan (Yang Hill Spring 阳陵泉 , GB 34, or gathering sinews): on the lateral aspect of the lower leg in the depression below the head of the fibula.

Indications: nausea, vomiting, contractions of the muscles, cramps or spasms, pain, and numbness in the legs.

• Dazhu (Big Reed 大杼 , BL 11, or gathering bones): on the upper back, level with the inferior border of the spine process of the first thoracic vertebra, 1.5 cun lateral of the midline.

Indications: cough, fever, headache, pain in the shoulder blade, and stiffness of the neck.

• Geshu (Diaphragm Back Transporting 膈俞 , BL 17, or gathering Blood): on the upper back, level with the inferior border of the spine process of the 7th thoracic vertebra, 1.5 cun lateral to the midline.

Indications: vomiting, hiccups, cough, tidal fever, and night sweating.

• Taiyuan (Greater Abyss 太渊 , LU 9, or gathering arteries and veins): on the palmar aspect of the wrist, in the depression at the radial end of the wrist crease, between the artery and tendon.

Indications: cough and asthma, mucus of blood, sore throat, palpitation, and pain in the chest and arm.

• Danzhong (Middle of Chest 膻中 , CV 17, or gathering Qi): parallel with the intercostal space of the fourth rib, at the front central line.

Indications: chronic cough, asthma, chest pain and pressure, and hiccups.

Chapter Eleven

Acupuncture

Acupuncture anesthesia is a technique that has achieved the effects of surgical anesthesia through the manipulation of acupuncture points. Many people first learned of acupuncture from there. In the early 1980s when I was in TCM medical college, we had internships in two phases, mid-term academic internships, and graduation internships. I met two highly-respected teachers in the acupuncture department during these two stages. At that time, acupuncture anesthesia was used to do surgery for appendicitis and for the sweat glands under the armpits. We observed the whole process in the operating room. Although it was not done by us, it made us feel great respect for acupuncturists. This was the beginning of my interest in meridian acupuncture. Much later, acupuncture and auricular acupoints cured my daughter's severe cough. I learned much meridian theory and clinical experience from Prof. Qiu Maoliang, chief doctor Sheng Canruo, chief doctor Cheng Zijun, and doctor Ding Duming (my brother-in-law). I followed their methods and used acupuncture to treat many internal conditions, which was the beginning of my frequent use of acupuncture for digestive and reproductive illnesses.

Over the last few years, there has been increasing evidence demonstrating the benefits of acupuncture and Chinese medicine during fertility treatments. A British Medical Acupuncture Society study concluded that three out of four randomized controlled trials revealed significantly higher pregnancy rates in the acupuncture group than in control groups.

What Is Acupuncture

Acupuncture is a system of medicine that follows the meridian energy distribution and direction of flow. It restores and supports health by the insertion of fine disposable needles gently into specific reaction points on the surface of the body. It varies according to different individuals and conditions. It also combines with methods of cupping, moxibustion, aromatherapy, and ear puncturing to suit specific conditions. These treatments stimulate or sedate the energy pathway and arouse the body's self-healing powers, restoring the overall energy balance.

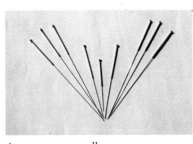

Acupuncture needles.

Acupuncture has the dual function of enhancing the mental and physiological functions of the human body and improving pathological changes by providing individualized treatment.

A Brief History of the Development of Acupuncture

Acupuncture and meridian theory originated in China and has existed for thousands of years.

Meridians are like an Internet running through the human body.

Acupoints are stations on the Internet. Qi and Blood are locomotives that pass through the stations. The "non-stop" sign is always displayed. Once Qi and Blood are stopped, doctors can only serve as network administrators.

The emergence of the book *The Yellow Emperor's Internal Canon of Medicine* indicates that the theoretical system of meridians and acupuncture and moxibustion was already formed at an early date. In this book, a complete meridian system has been established, with twelve regular meridians, fifteen collaterals, twelve branches, tendons, muscle, and the skin of the meridians. The eight extraordinary vessels are also included. There is also a very specific discussion of meridian diseases and their treatment. The meridian theory was formed and developed from the long-term practice of life and the accumulated practical experience of treatment. Its guide and all clinical techniques were also enriched and improved from repeated processes.

Nine Needles is an early record of acupuncture treatment and is mentioned in five places in *The Spiritual Pivot* (*Ling Shu*) from *The Yellow Emperor's Internal Canon of Medicine*. The book refers to needles of different sizes and lengths (diameter and length of the needle body) combined with the needle shape to treat different parts of body's illness and properties (skin, muscle, tendon, etc.) of the disease.

The needles directly reach some of the diseased areas. The stimulation can be moderate inside the lesion to achieve pain relief, reduce numbness, and any foreign body sensation (burning, an ant row climbing, etc.), promoting Qi movement to expel swelling, recover dysfunctions, and other purposes.

Huang Fumi's acupuncture monograph *The Systematic Classic of Acupuncture and Moxibustion* (also known as *The Yellow Emperor's Systematic Classic of Acupuncture and Moxibustion in Three Parts*) was published in the Jin dynasty (266–420). It is a deeper, wider systematic acupuncture theory system and is convenient for the clinical application of acupuncture treatment. It was at this time that acupuncture treatment became an independent clinical branch, which had a far-reaching influence on the development of acupuncture and moxibustion. In the Tang (618–907) and Song (960–1279) dynasties, this book was listed as the main work of acupuncturists for studying and testing for medical practice.

Wang Weiyi of the Northern Song dynasty (960–1127) compiled *Illustrated Classic of Acupoints on the Bronze Figure* (abbrev. *Classic of the Bronze Figure* or *The Bronze Figure*), where the meridians and acupoints were discussed and 354 acupoints were examined. Two different models were illustrated in *Classic of Acupoints on the Bronze Figure*, including all meridians and acupuncture points on the surface of body, which were also cast for study and examination.

The Ming dynasty was a prosperous period in the development of acupuncture and moxibustion, and there was a large number of acupuncture books published, in particular, *The Great Compendium of Acupuncture and Moxibustion* was written by Yang Jishi. Dr. Yang gathered results from acupuncture before the Ming dynasty, summing up the clinical experience that was rich in content. It remains the main reference book for subsequent students to study acupuncture.

After 1949, acupuncture developed very rapidly. Acupuncture branches are widely established in Chinese medicine hospitals and modern medical hospitals. In the early 1960s, the Shanghai College of Traditional Chinese Medicine established an acupuncture, moxibustion, and Tuina section to train acupuncturists and Tuinaists, which was listed as a national formal training program. Today, around 25 universities and colleges in China have established acupuncture-moxibustion and Tuina colleges or departments.

Acupuncture Functions

The main roles of acupuncture proposed by modern research are:
- Regulating the coordinated correlation between the nervous system and muscles.
- Two-way adjustment of the functions of the visceral system.
- Promoting blood circulation and lymphatic flow, accelerating secretion of chemicals and improving threshold of feeling, regulating and balancing the relationship between the nerves, immune, and endocrine functions.

The main roles of acupuncture proposed by TCM are:
- Adjusting the balance between Qi and Blood, Yin and Yang.
- Smoothing and dredging channels and collaterals.

• Enhancing the body's disease resistance and assisting the body's defensive function (*fu zheng*), eliminating the factors that cause disease (*qu xie*).

Acupuncture Methods

Since acupuncture is a licensed practice, I will only introduce here some general information for your reference. There are two methods of inserting a needle into an acupoint:

1. Finger Pressure Needling

The thumb or index finger of the left hand is pressed on the side of the acupuncture point. The needle held in the right hand is placed close to the left hand, then inserted into the acupoint. This method is easy to operate and accurate in positioning, and there is less discomfort for the patient when inserting the needle. It is most commonly used in clinical practice.

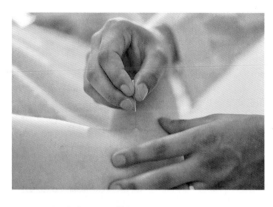

Finger pressure needling.

2. Quick Needling

Depending on the size of the needle used, prepare metal tubes of different sizes to make the needle 0.5 to 1 cun longer than the metal tube. For example, use a 1.5-cun needle and use a 1.4 to 1.45-cun metal tube. A trocar needle can also be purchased. Replace the hands with metal tubes to place on the chosen acupoint, tap the needle in or bounce it in from the tube into the acupuncture point. When this is done, remove the metal tube, lifting it upwards.

Acupuncture can also be combined with different techniques:

Hand stimulation: Making the needle go up or down, from the superficial to the deeper part of the body, or twisting the needle in at different speeds by the practitioner's hands.

Electronic stimulator: Using an electrode sheet (piece) or needles, collecting electro-acupuncture instrument clamps to click into the two electrode sheets or two needles, then determining the frequency and speed, turning on the electronic stimulator to the minimum response level. Continue for 20 to 25 minutes.

Moxibustion or warming: For Cold or Damp conditions, we can combine acupuncture with moxibustion or magnetic rays. For instance, when treating a painful shoulder (frozen shoulder), we can combine moxibustion or infrared rays to the Jianyu point (LI 15) and the Jianliao point (TE 14).

"Feel the Qi" and the Curative Effects of Acupuncture

After the complete insertion of a needle, the TCM doctor will use techniques to make you feel certain sensations. Some feel heavy and relaxed, while others feel a little bit full and tender. One may even feel a small tingling or some heat. This feeling indicates that you are harnessing your positive energy in order to remove the blocked energy. It is believed that if one has this kind of feeling, one will respond to the acupuncture treatment better, meaning that after stimulating some part of your body, your energy could respond, the blockage could be opened easily, and this acupuncture method is well suited to your condition.

The function of the meridians is called Meridian Qi, which is invisible, but its conduction and induction can be expressed through many pathological changes and feedback from the treatment process. In the process of acupuncture, if the patient can "feel the Qi," or feels "the Qi move," it means the Qi makes you feel sore, fullness, or a minor twitch. After being transmitted from the limbs to the trunk, the Meridian Qi tends to the diseased area. For example, if the heart has problem, the needle sensation from different meridian points are transmitted from limbs to the chest and abdomen, all tending to focus on the heart, also known as *qi zhi bing suo* 气至病所 (Meridian Qi reaches the diseased location). It can be expressed as adjustments to many pathological conditions. When some acupuncture points show two-way regulation after the needle is inserted, it is also known as adaptation to the original effect, which means that if there is a palpitation, we place a needle in the Neiguan point (PC 6) to slow down the heartbeat. If there is a slow pulse, we place a needle in the Neiguan point to increase the heartbeat. We can make an original hyperactive condition inhibited, or an original inhibition excited. In this way, the Yin and Yang of the viscera are coordinated, and the functions of the whole body are adjusted to make it harmonious and balanced.

The technique of "feeling Qi" on a distant point can also clear acute blockage and open skin pores and muscle nodules to reduce acute pain. For example, the US Air Force uses ear reflection points to do ear acupuncture to treat pain in the field. This pain can include headaches or sore neck and shoulders, for which the acupuncture has amazing results. Pain in the head, neck, and shoulders can be treated with strong auricular pressure as well.

Common Acupuncture Categories
Fine needle acupuncture suits people who are afraid of needles.

Thick, bigger needles (*xiao zhen dao*) are used to treat long-term, chronic pain located in deeper tendons.

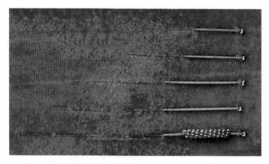

Different sizes of needle.

Bee needle acupuncture uses bee stings on the patient's skin, combined with traditional acupuncture points. Bee poison has a high concentration of biological and pharmacological components. The bee toxin liquid has anti-bacteria, anti-inflammation, and anti-high lipid components. Bee stings stimulating the reaction point can increase blood circulation and speed up the local tissue metabolism. A polypeptide found in bee poison has a certain effect for some nervous systems and can promote the secretion of pituitary adrenaline (but be sure to avoid sensitive or allergic reactions). Bee needle acupuncture treatment can be applied for pain, rheumatism, or rheumatoid arthritis.

Acupuncture Precautions

You may occasionally undergo minor bruises and local allergic reactions during acupuncture. A small piece of cyanosis can appear in the body part, which generally does not have to be treated, and will resolve itself within three to five days.

On an empty stomach or with excessive fatigue and mental stress, it is not advisable to apply acupuncture. If you have symptoms such as dizziness, pain, nausea, or others during the acupuncture treatment, it is an adverse reaction to the acupuncture. You should immediately tell the doctor about the symptoms and stop the treatment to prevent further discomfort. If you have low blood pressure, hypoglycemia, excessive weakness, and nervous tension, you should also be cautious.

Do not insert the needle too deep in the points near the chest, back, or abdomen near internal organs. Use small and medium needles and an oblique method. Please keep your body in a stable position during treatment as well.

When the patient is more than two months pregnant, acupuncture for associated pain, vomiting, and other symptoms should avoid specific parts and specific acupoints such as the Hegu point (LI 4), Sanyinjiao point (SP 6), Jianjing point (GB 21). If the patient has had a miscarriage, it is best not to undergo acupuncture.

Do not insert the needle on skin where there are ulcers, moles, or other lesions. If one has a tendency toward serious bleeding, such as hemophilia, do not conduct acupuncture.

Chapter Twelve

Moxibustion and Related Warmth Therapies

According to TCM's understanding of pathogeny, there are many illnesses related to Coldness in the environment. This includes both climate and artificial cold, such as excessive use of air conditioning indoors or working in a cold environment, as in jobs where one may be exposed to chillers/freezers, or even ingesting foods that are too cold or frozen. All of these can cause certain illnesses.

In addition, as people age, their body energy movement slows down. The body produces less Yang energy, allowing Coldness to be generated from the inside.

Both external and internal causes of Coldness in Chinese medicine and culture can lead to a large range of aches and discomfort. There's an old Chinese saying, *han cong jiao xia qi* 寒从脚下起 , meaning that Coldness enters the body through the bottom of the feet, which reminds people to protect the feet so as not to let the Coldness penetrate the body, especially during the cold seasons. Another saying, *yin bu shi chi han* 饮不使齿寒 , means that one should not drink liquids that cause the teeth to feel cold, reminding us to protect our body by refraining from icy drinks. *Bai lu shen bu lu, han lu zu bu lu* 白露身不露，寒露足不露 is another traditional saying, meaning that once the White Dew solar term is upon us around September 8 every year, we should not have too much skin exposed, and once the Cold Dew solar term arrives around October 8, we should not walk around barefoot. Wearing socks to protect feet from Coldness has been connected to boosting the immune system, especially the upper respiratory tract. If people already have chronic problems such as arthritis or asthma, Cold Dew is the time that the symptoms can easily arise or attack again.

What Is Moxibustion

Moxibustion is a very common practice in TCM therapy. Using a naturally Warm property ingredient and burning it can transfer the heat and warmth through the skin to make our body stronger. There is a double receiving factor. First, chemically it comes from the properties of mugwort leaf, and second, physically it comes from the warmth of the fire. Burning of the mugwort leaf is a method that has been practiced for generations and grown from practical experience.

Moxa has been designed to help harmonize or treat these Cold factors. It is made from mugwort (argy wormwood) leaf. Mugwort comes from the Asteraceae family (Latin name: folium artemisiae argyi). Through a specific technique, the leaves are made into soft, fine pieces. The TCM doctor usually wraps these in paper, rolling them into a long cigar shape. Another method is to form them into a cone shape and place it on top of a piece of ginger or garlic to be burned over a patient's body. The smoke will produce a warming effect on the body. Usually the doctor will perform moxibustion in

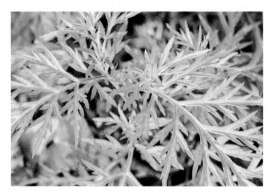

Mugwort leaf.

different forms on people with Yang energy deficiency, Qi deficiency, or with too much Cold accumulated in the body. Moxibustion can also be combined with acupuncture.

Another use of moxibustion is for people with weak constitutions who do not have any illness, but use it for prevention and to strengthen the body. Moxibustion can help regulate blood circulation and improve digestion and energy. Usually people will use it on the body specifically on the Zusanli point (ST 36) during the first ten days of the lunar month for three consecutive months.

A Brief History of the Development of Moxibustion

Warmth therapy started when our ancestors discovered fire and started exploring different temperatures to help ease bodily discomfort. Three articles on meridian moxibustion were recorded in the silk manuscripts unearthed from Mawangdui (a tomb dating from the Western Han dynasty, 206 BC–AD 25) in Changsha, Hunan Province of China in 1973, which shows that moxibustion originates from ancient times, earlier than the period of the book *The Yellow Emperor's Internal Canon of Medicine*.

Later, the practice of moxibustion was mixed with other herbs. Today, you can purchase pure mugwort leaves, moxa, or mugwort mixed with other herbs, which is more like a prescription, customized according to your needs and targeting certain parts of the body through the skin. The records of moxibustion were written in *The Yellow Emperor's Internal Canon of Medicine*, which says that moxibustion is good for treating Cold conditions. This was followed by Zhang Zhongjing's *Treatise on Exogenous Febrile Disease*, which likewise notes that Cold can trigger many kinds of diseases and advises using moxibustion to help stimulate the warmth in certain areas of the body. In the Jin dynasty, Doctor Ge strongly advised moxibustion to be combined with acupuncture. He created 109 formulas, 99 of which included moxa, and he helped solidify the use of moxa in TCM. In the Tang dynasty, the well-known doctor Sun Simiao (581–682) wrote a book called *Important Formulas Worth a Thousand Gold Pieces* (*Qian Jin Yao Fang*). He is considered the first doctor who thought moxa could help in the prevention of many illnesses.

Warmth therapy opened new ideas for dealing with acute injuries, old aches, or circulation problems. When other treatments do not seem to work, sometimes using moxa can have seemingly miraculous results. Ming dynasty doctor Li Chan, in his book *Introduction to Medicine*, claims that "if medicine cannot treat your issue fast enough and acupuncture needles cannot reach it, then you must use moxibustion." Internationally, more people are familiar with using cold therapy, such as ice packs (or a bag of frozen peas) to treat fever and inflammation, but Chinese people recommend that in certain situations, it is better to try warmer remedies.

Moxibustion Techniques

Through the process of burning mugwort leaves, antioxidants are released and with the heat from the fire, the pores on the skin open to become more receptive to these antioxidants. Using moxa on meridians and acupoints is even better. These areas on the body are more sensitive to moxa. Regardless of whether you have hyper or hypo conditions, a deficiency or an excess, moxibustion can bring you back to natural balance, producing a double immunity regulation effect. Above all, the moxibustion technique is explained as first being a warm method, and second, the properties of the mugwort leaf (or combination with other herbs) can be absorbed chemically by the human body. Finally, its overall response, like opening skin pores, increasing external immunity.

Application of Moxibustion

There are many methods for applying moxibustion. Here, I will mainly introduce the simpler methods, suitable for home application to help regularly strengthen your health. Different methods target

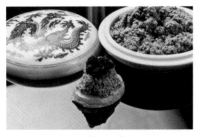

Ginger-Separated Moxibustion.

different conditions and will bring about different results.

Ginger-Separated Moxibustion: Cut out a round piece of ginger about 2 centimeters thick and 3 centimeters in diameter and place it on the acupoints. If the patient has a cold stomach, place the ginger on the Zhongwan point (CV 12), then place the fine pieces of moxa (mugwort leaves) on top of the ginger. Light the moxa pieces with a match or lighter until it burns out, then repeat the process again for a second and third time, depending on the condition being treated. Sometimes, the doctor may choose two or three points to treat at the same time, burning at these points together, repeating three to five times. Garlic-Separated Moxibustion and Sea Salt-Separated Moxibustion are similar, but using garlic or sea salt rather than ginger. Using sea salt can produce both opposite yet complementary effects.

Moxa stick: There are two kinds of moxa sticks. One is made from pure mugwort leaves and the other is mixed with 8 to 10 other herbs. For beginners, we recommend using pure mugwort leaves as opposed to a mix, because some people may be intolerant or sensitive to the other herbs. Pregnant patients can be treated with moxa sticks. For example, for women in the last trimester (above 30 weeks), if the baby's position is not ideal, with the head facing up, TCM doctors will usually advise the pregnant woman to apply moxibustion on the Bladder Meridian point Zhiyin (BL 67), in a motion called Sparrow-Pecking Moxibustion. The moxibustion is performed with a movement like a bird pecking. Each time, this point will be warmed for 8 to 10 minutes, according to the person's condition, one to two times a day. After three to four days, the baby's head will usually turn down towards the uterus opening. We advise pregnant woman to try these five times, but many people have success with just three applications. One of my students learned this method in Shanghai. She moved to Korea, where there was no moxa, so she asked if she could use a hair dryer. Each time she used the dryer to blow at the Zhiyin point (BL 67) for 8 to 10 minutes. After a few times, the baby's head turned. This happened with electrical heat, which also did the trick. If people dislike the moxa smell or do not have access to moxa, electronically stimulated heating methods might work. Another method is to move the moxa stick in a clock-wise circular motion (*hui xuan fa*), which is used quite often to treat menstruation issues. If someone is menstruating for ten days or longer with pink leucorrhea, we will use moxa on the 7th day on the Yinbai point (SP 1) of the Spleen Meridian on the foot for three treatments to help the menstruation shorten to a more normal range.

Moxa machine: This is a combination of electricity and traditional moxa. This equipment is considered easier to use for some, and it produces less smell than the traditional moxa stick. For example, if you have a stiff neck, you might choose to use the machine on your Triple Energizer or *Sanjiao* Meridian to help. This method is the easiest to use.

Moxa box: This box consists of three parts, one box made from bamboo with holes, and moxa holder with a small piece of moxa. We light the moxa, then place it on the holder in the box. We then close the box and put the box's hole over the part of the body that feels discomfort. If a patient has knee pain, we would put the box over the knee area and repeat this process three times. For people who have aversion to cold or Yang deficiency, we can also regularly use this in topical cold area. Recently some doctors have been applying moxibustion to cancer patients to help ease their pain and protect the patient's immune functions with no side effects. This method does not require electricity.

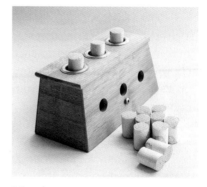

Moxa box.

Things to Consider

Select high quality mugwort: Choose good quality brands and mugwort that is more than a year old. If it is too young, it may not be as effective.

When using moxa at home, be very careful, with one hand holding the moxa stick. Pay attention to what motions you use and how big the moxa cone is, and try experimenting with the ones that give you most comfort.

Moxa is usually used to treat people with Cold and deficiencies. If you also have Hot tendencies, it is better not to use moxa for too long or in excess, in order to avoid disturbing or weakening Blood or losing liquid. Be careful not to burn yourself. Today, smokeless moxa is available. Remember to take in enough water after moxibustion, so as not to lose density in the blood.

When Not to Use Moxibustion

Do not use moxibustion if you have high fever, severe high blood pressure, are in the late stages of an infectious disease, cough up blood, have severe vomiting, a family history of anemia, or extremely heavy menstruation. Generally, if you are menstruating and feeling fine, we would not recommend moxibustion.

Avoid applying moxibustion near the big arteries on the skin surface, mucus membrane areas such as the mouth, anus, vagina, or to the face, neck, heart area.

Do not use moxibustion if you are suffering from severe exhaustion and internal damage from accidents.

Related Warmth Therapies and Treatments

There are many other treatments, such as heat patches, which can help with Cold-related conditions. Hot water bottle bags or copper bottles and warm packs that you can keep under your clothes can also help. Essential oils can help generate warmth in the body, such as safflower oil (红花油) or warming Tiger Balm (万金 油). One can rub the oil over the painful area to warm it up and boost circulation. We can use warming Tiger Balm to help with a baby's cough, rubbing it on the Kidney Meridian point Yongquan (KI 1) on the bottom of the feet. Another method is putting a 1-cm-thick and 2-cm-in-diameter piece of ginger on the bottom of baby's feet, keeping it in place with plastic wrap or a bandage overnight, which helps many babies below one year old recover quickly from an asthmatic or productive cough.

If you have warts, you can also treat them by using Tiger Balm combined with moxibustion or air from a hair dryer to help soften or shrink the warts. It is recommended that this be done twice a day for seven consecutive days.

Therefore, there are several methods you can try in addition to or instead of moxibustion. You can use a hair dryer to warm local parts for 3 to 5 minutes and massage certain parts of your body for 20 minutes. After drying, apply saffron oil on an acupoint, then put a special magnetic coin with a plastic stick cover that can help further alleviate discomfort, such as aches and pains in muscles and joints. Another method is to blend some spices like chili, cloves, and cinnamon into powder form and mix it with ointment. Applying this mixture on the rib area can help alleviate rib pain. Applying it to the abdominal Stomach Meridian acupoints or on the belly button can greatly reduce bloating and diarrhea. You may also use different herbs, including mugwort and safflower, to soak the feet in hot water. Hot water with different herbs can also increase blood circulation. These are all various warmth therapies to help to alleviate pain and discomfort stemming from Cold.

Chapter Thirteen
Tuina Manipulation and Chinese Massage

I have been teaching and practicing Chinese medicine in Shanghai for more than 24 years. Every year, I contact many domestic and foreign customers who want to use Chinese medicine to prevent and treat diseases. If I ask them, "Do you know much about TCM? Which is the most common therapy in TCM? Have you ever used TCM therapy?" Most domestic friends know more about herbal medicines and functional foods, while people from other countries and regions are more familiar with Chinese massage (Tuina).

Touch between lovers has a special power to enhance happy chemical secretion. Embracing and touching each other can calm us down and help our system to heal.

Touch between a professional masseur and a patient can offer more benefits, if both are suited to each other. Massage performed by a TCM doctor is called Tuina manipulation. Cranial therapy and foot reflexology belong in this category.

The Twelve Skin Zones

The entire surface of your face and body skin is divided into 12 zones, which are related to the 12 meridians (also see page 100). By noticing issues or problems within specific division, it is possible to know which organ system may be out of balance.

For instance, you may notice patches of dryness, varicose or spider veins, or pigmentation in certain regions. Taking note of where these conditions regularly appear can help with diagnosis. You can use the "12 skin zones" theory as a reference. Your practitioner might treat the meridians related to these zones with acupuncture, massage, and acupressure.

The heart system controls the Heart, Small Intestine, Pericardium, and *Sanjiao* Meridians. The pericardium is the outer membrane of the heart, and its meridian connects with the *Sanjiao* Meridian. According to this theory, if a skin condition is found in any of these areas, you might look at treating the heart system first.

The lung system controls the lung and large intestine zones. If acne appears on the side of the nose and upper chest area, which is more related to lung system, you might need to focus on your lungs.

The liver system controls the liver and gall bladder zones, the spleen system controls the spleen and stomach divisions, and the kidney system controls the kidney and bladder divisions.

What Is Tuina

Tuina is a kind of Chinese massage, a form of hand manipulation. In Chinese *tui* means push, and *na* means grab or take. It is a therapeutic method based on the meridian theory, an integral component of TCM.

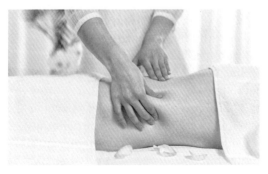

Tuina massage.

A Brief History of the Development of Tuina Therapy

Massage was first recorded in the *Yellow Emperor's Internal Canon of Medicine*. It notes that "when the body experiences repeated fear or panic, the channels are blocked. The body will feel numb and should be treated by massage combined with herbal wine." Zhang Zhongjing, a medical practitioner of the Eastern Han dynasty, was the first to propose the *gaomo* treatment in his book *Treatise on Cold Damage and Miscellaneous Diseases*. *Gaomo* treatment is the use of herbal ointment in Chinese massage to achieve a combined double effect of manipulation and medicine, which broadens its application and elevates the therapeutic effect.

The Sui (581–618) and Tang dynasties were a flourishing age for Chinese massage. A massage branch was set up in the office of the imperial physicians of the Tang dynasty, and the masseur was classified as massage doctors, masseurs, and massage workers. Massage doctors taught students how to combine hand pushing and abdominal breathing together to treat illness and injuries, indicating the prosperous teaching and practice of Chinese massage at that time. *Important Formulas Worth a Thousand Gold Pieces*, written by Sun Simiao in the 7th century, further developed *gaomo* into the prescriptions and drugs of massage therapy, especially as applied to children.

After 1949, the scope of massage included treating internal, external, gynecology, pediatrics, and ENT disorders, among others. At the same time, meticulous work on the history of massage was carried out, and the mechanism of treatment through massage was discussed and many books were published.

At present, acupuncture combined with Chinese massage is one of the three fields of learning in TCM. Tuina plays an important role in many aspects, such as medical services, rehabilitation, and health care.

The Mechanism of Chinese Tuina Massage

There are three main areas in Chinese massage. The first is regulating Yin and Yang, the second is regulating the function of channels and collaterals, Qi, Blood, and internal organs, and the third is recovery of the function of tendons, bones, and joints.

These functional principles of Chinese Tuina massage are very similar to the principles of acupuncture. The difference is that one uses needles and the other is done by hand. If people are afraid of needles, Chinese massage will be a good alternative, especially for children, very weak people, or the elderly.

Chinese Massage Procedures and the Methods

I will focus on certain types of discomfort to introduce you some common Chinese massage procedures and methods. In particular, I will share some information on how to help babies reduce certain aches and discomfort.

Eye massage. If performed regularly, eye massages can really improve the appearance of the eyes, reduce wrinkles, and lift the eyes. Massages can be done with or without facial oil.

First, sit still with your ankles, knees, hips all at right angles, or lie down in a comfortable position.

Second, find the Cuanzhu point (BL 2) using the tips of your thumbs. Massage in circular motions 32 times clockwise and 32 times counterclockwise.

Third, inside the depression against the bridge of the nose, in line with the inner eye, find the Jingming point (BL 1) to massage. Repeat the procedure of massaging the point in a total of 64 circular movements.

Fourth, the Sibai point (ST 2) is just below your eyes (in line with your eyeballs on the peaks of the cheekbones). Find the small depression there and use your index fingers to repeat the massage procedure. You can rest your thumbs on the jaw as you massage.

Finally, place the thumbs on both sides of the temple, namely Taiyang point (EX-HN 5) and use the outer edge of the forefingers to massage across the eyebrows (starting from the inside out and moving in straight lines). Alternate between the top of the eyebrows

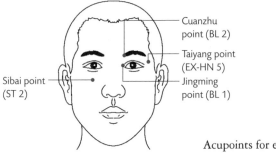

Acupoints for eye massage.

and the bone under the eyes (also from the inside out), then follow the same path to massage in small circular movements.

Digital pushing method for migraines. This is a basic manipulation. Stretch the thumb with the fingers open, then push with the tip of the thumb on Taiyang point (EX-HN 5) at an angle of 90 degree clockwise for 20 seconds. The same method can also be applied on the back of neck at the Fengchi point (GB 20) to relieve headaches or stress.

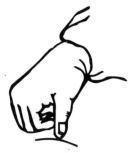

Digital pushing method.

Spine pinching is a simple and effective form of folk rehabilitative therapy which focuses on manipulation of the musculoskeletal system, especially the spine. The main spine pinching treatment technique involves manual therapy, especially on both sides of the spine. It overlaps with other manual-therapy approaches, such as osteopathy and physical therapy. For babies

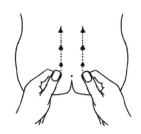

Spine pinching starts here.

with a weak constitution, you can use the spine pinching method from both sides of the tailbone all the way up to both sides of the neck. Do this once a day for about three months to complete a course. If the condition is more complicated, a longer period of treatment may be needed or combined with the use of herbs. For children, it is mainly effective for dyspepsia and digestive disorders (loss of appetite, vomiting, abdominal distension, diarrhea, and constipation), infantile malnutrition, nocturia, and insomnia. For adults, it has proven effective for insomnia, drowsiness, acute and chronic gastritis, acute and chronic enteritis, chronic hepatitis, neurasthenia, hypertension, lumbago, and other disorders.

The spine pinching treatment involves several steps. The patient should first assume a prone position for the treatment.

• Use both hands and keep the hands loose, with the thumbs below the four fingers. Then press the skin with the thumbs facing toward the head.

• The fingers pinch the skin as if rolling along the spinal column from the coccyx upwards to the Dazhui point (GV 14) of the cervical vertebrae. Repeat the procedure three times. (For severe cases, the movements may be supplemented by spine pinching of the Bladder Meridians along both sides of the spinal column. In order to achieve favorable results, the physician may need to repeat an additional three times).

• Select pressure points connected to the symptoms. For instance, the Pishu point (BL 20) should be massaged to treat dyspepsia, the Xinshu point (BL 15) for insomnia, and the Shenshu (BL 23) for lumbago and hypertension. Pinch and lift the skin forcefully for three times for one to two minutes.

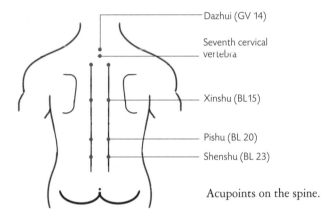

Dazhui (GV 14)

Seventh cervical vertebra

Xinshu (BL15)

Pishu (BL 20)

Shenshu (BL 23)

Acupoints on the spine.

Let's review six essential points:

• The patient can receive treatment daily or every other day.

• For pinching movements, ensure that both hands use an even amount of strength. The skin being pinched should be of appropriate thickness, and ensure that the pinching action is tight. Generally speaking, skin of 0.5 to 1 cm in thickness is suitable for this treatment.

• For loss of appetite, massage before eating a meal. For dyspepsia, distension of the abdomen, and stuffy chest, massage after a meal.

• For insomnia and nocturia, a spine massage before going to bed will aid in sleep patterns.

• During summer, if the back is sweaty, first dry it with a towel, then apply some talcum powder to prevent slippery skin.

• Tuina is not useful for skin infection.

Chapter Fourteen
Cupping Therapy

At the Rio Summer Olympics, the cupping marks over American swimmer Michael Phelps' body sparked the attention of Chinese netizens. This kind of green, non-drug therapy has long been widely used in China and has been recognized by foreign countries and many professional athletes, sparking heated discussion. In China, in the hottest part of summer, you may encounter many people in the street who have can-shaped prints on their bodies, arms, and necks. This kind of cupping therapy, which is popular and widely sought after by the public, is called the new "natural therapy" of the 21st century because of its wide application range, good curative effect, affordability, ease of use, and absence of side effects.

In fact, cupping is not new, and it is not even unique to China. Cupping therapy was also popular in ancient Greek and Roman times. In ancient Western medicine, cupping was called cup suction. In a doctor's diary from Babylon, we find the image of the health god Nuuta or Adar holding cupping equipment. A horn cup and glass cup were the main tools used in cup suction. In the 19th century, new instruments were introduced that combined syringes and suction cups. The African continent, Japan, and India also have records of such extractive therapies.

What Is Cupping and Its Function
In China, cupping uses cups as a tool, applying fire, pumping, and other methods to eliminate the oxygen in the cup to generate negative pressure. The underlying tissue is raised into the cup, so the cup suctions on the surface of the meridian points. People choose cupping therapy for many reasons, including helping with pain, enhancing blood circulation, promoting lymphatic flow, and releasing stuck fascia (connective tissue). Through stimulation, it also achieves the effects of relieving Phlegm and Cold, reducing swelling, and strengthening the body. Overall, it promotes healing, prevents illness, reduces stress, and brings about relaxation and a sense of well-being.

A Brief History of the Development of Cupping Therapy
Cupping therapy has a long history in China. The first records of cupping methods can be traced back to the Western Han dynasty

in the 3rd century BC, when it was used as a common method for surgery. For instance, in the *Fifty-Two Diseases*, written in the Spring and Autumn period and Warring States period (770–221 BC), there are records concerning the "horn method," which is similar to the cupping therapy of later generations, where it is called "suction tube therapy" and is mainly used for the surgical treatment of sores, releasing blood and pus.

It is only in the Tang dynasty volume, Wang Shu's *The Secrets of the Outer Taiwan*, that we find an official description of the cupping method as a therapy. In the Song and Ming dynasties, the applications of cupping was extended to medical diseases. For example, it was used to treat chronic coughs and was used with the combination of syndrome differentiation and bamboo cups. The "boiling bamboo cup method" applied the boiling of traditional medicine bamboo cups to improve its curative effects. In the Qing dynasty, Wu Qian recorded the method of cupping combined with herbs and acupuncture treatment in *Golden Mirror of the Medical Tradition (Yi Zong Jin Jian)*, which is still in use today.

After 1949, with the inheritance and development of TCM, cupping therapy was applied to clinical subjects such as internal, external, women and children's medicine, and bone injuries, skin, ENT, and other areas. Its content and utilization were recorded and established in many monographs, establishing the academic status of cupping. The course of study of the modern Chinese medicine university discusses the cupping method after presenting the moxibustion method. With the popularization of clinical practices, the materials of the cups and the cupping methods have been improved, while the scope of treatment has gradually expanded. It has become one of the popular treatments for acupuncture and moxibustion departments. It has also been favored by many foreign patients and is applicable to a variety of internal surgical diseases. It is very popular in family health care.

Functions of Cupping Therapy

The negative pressure generated during cupping has the effects of opening the pores, dehumidification, weight loss, and dispelling Wind and Coldness, and helps to reduce body discomfort and restore physical functions. For example, when children are suffering from rhinitis or otitis after swimming, you can select the Fengchi (GB 20) or Waiguan point (TE 5) for cupping to dispel Coldness and Wind, soothe the sinuses, and relieve blockage of the nose and ears, which could be achieved through suction on the acupoints to regulate the meridians, Qi and Blood and regulate the internal organs to achieve a well-balanced status. For adults suffering from pharyngitis or bronchitis, cupping along the Bladder Meridian such as the Dazhui point (GV 14) or Feishu point (BL 13) can excrete sputum and relieve coughs, accelerating the recovery process. Cupping can also adjust damaged tissue and reduce pain. For example, for a frozen shoulder, cupping on the points of Jianzhen (SI 9), Jianliao (TE 14), Jianyu (LI 15) on the shoulders can relieve swelling and pain.

Materials for Cups

There are three main types of cups, each with its own advantages and disadvantages.

Bamboo cups, which are made from bamboo tubes. The advantages to this kind of cup is that its materials are easy to procure, economical, easy to manufacture, light, handy, and sturdy. The disadvantages are that it cracks easily after heating, causing it to leak air.

Glass cups, which are made of thick glass, can also be replaced by a wide-mouthed glass bottle. The advantage of this type is that the cups are transparent. During use, the acupoints on the skin can be observed to determine the extent of the congestion, making it flexible for treatment and easy to disinfect. Its disadvantage is that it is easy to break.

Pumping cups are made of PVC plastic or silicone cups. By extracting oxygen from the cup, it can be suctioned from the surface of the acupoints. The advantages include being observable, operable, easy to carry, and that it is transparent. It is the most ideal cup for families and self-learners. As

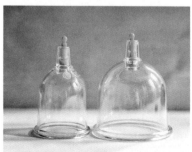

Pumping cups.

we go into details for the specific cupping methods, I will use the pumping cup as an example.

Cupping Methods

Take 3 to 5 medium to large sized PVC suction cups, connect the suction cylinder to the cups, and pull out 3 to 5 times. Apply a medium amount of negative pressure during the initial cupping process. As the number of times you apply suction increases, you can gradually increase the negative pressure. After that, leave the cups for 8 to 12 minutes. The practitioner can adjust the treatment time for people with sensitive skin. The practitioner should observe the acupoints closely, and when congestion occurs on the acupoints, the suction cups should be removed.

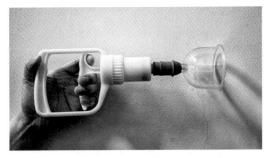

Using PVC suction cups.

There is another kind of hot spring hydro-cupping method. It involves first putting small bamboo cups in a hot spring pool (or a well), then using a strainer to retrieve the cups, shaking off water droplets, and immediately attaching the cups to the meridian points to ensure they can suck on skin. This method is part of the medicine canister cupping method. A variety of TCM herbs can be placed into a cloth bag after they are boiled for 10 to 15 minutes with the bamboo cups, then used to attach the medicine bamboo cups onto the affected parts. Medicine cupping produces multiple affects, such as warming and mechanical and herbal percutaneous absorption. It can be used for treating rheumatism pain, asthma, chronic gastritis, and other ailments.

In order to utilize medical cupping treatments to cure muscle rheumatism, you can:

• Choose acupoints, selecting 3 to 4 Ashi points (trigger points).

- Herbs: 40 grams each of chaenomeles lagenaria koidz (*mu gua*), caulis spatholobi (*ji xue teng*), honeysuckle twig (*reng dong teng*), mugwort (*ai ye*).
- Boil those herbs with small bamboo cups for 15 minutes, using suction on the skin to pull tissue into the cups, then keep the cups in place for 12 minutes.

Cupping therapy is an independent treatment method based on the fundamental theories of TCM, influenced by the theory of Yin and Yang and the theory of viscera and meridians. Although it only stimulates local areas or meridian acupoints, with its simple operation and quick effect, it can be combined with both herbs and acupuncture. It is able to be sensed through the meridians and trigger local and even systemic reactions, thereby adjusting the body function and allowing unobstructed meridians to achieve the goals of regulating Qi and Blood, balancing Yin and Yang, and promoting blood circulation, which can also dispel Coldness, remove edema, and relax the muscles.

The De-Cupping Method

For suction cups, as long as the top cover is opened, the air can be let into the tank. In order to de-cup the glass jars or bamboo cans, first hold the cups with your left hand, press local skin with the right thumb or forefinger from the side of the tank to let air into the cup, and it can be easily removed.

Conditions Suitable for Cupping

When you have a cough, stomach pain, vomiting, abdominal pain, diarrhea, or other similar symptoms, you may try cupping. Preventive care and treatment of joints, muscles, tendons, sore neck, and shoulder syndromes can also be treated through cupping.

If you use glass jars or bamboo cans for cupping, you must use 80% to 95% alcohols to ignite and use the flash-fire method for cupping. If you want to learn the flash-fire method, I recommend you attend a training course in a medical institution.

Cupping during the hottest days of summer, in addition to preventive cupping, can cure winter diseases. Cupping also has diagnostic and anti-toxic functions, preventing people from catching cold during the summer. This method includes arranging 6 to 8 cups on the back vertically and horizontally, sometimes accompanied by needles. First, apply acupuncture in certain acupoints, then apply the cupping method around the center of the needles. This is called the needle through cupping method.

Identifying Certain Conditions from the Related Marks

Generally speaking, after 8 to 12 minutes of cupping, people will show a fresh pink-red color, red or deep red color, or light or dark purple color on the cupped skin. If it is fresh pink-red color, it means the condition is quite mild. After the color disappears, the pain or aching experienced in the body should be reduced.

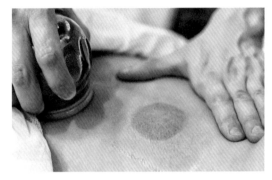

Cupping mark.

If it is blood red or deep red color, it means this person has a Hot body condition and the cupping marks will turn pale in 3 to 5 days. In order to speed up the effects of treatment, one can repeat the cupping therapy, combined with eating cooling foods.

If the color is light purple, it means there is some stagnation in the body. If it is darker purple, that means there is Cold Dampness in the meridians or toxins are blocked in the blood. This requires more sessions for treatment and specific foods and herbs to remove the Cold-Dampness or to help speed up the blood circulation.

If you feel light and comfortable after cupping and the mark recovers quite quickly, it means you are suited to cupping treatment. Even you do not have any complaints, it is advisable for you to do cupping in the hottest days of summer as a detoxing method.

Precautions

You should choose the appropriate position and select the acupoints on body parts where there is relatively thick muscle. Remove the hair around the related areas prior to cupping. For patients with thinner or sensitive skin, leave the cups for 8 minutes or less. For patients with healthy skin, leave the cups for 10 minutes. The cupping time can be gradually prolonged based on the situation.

If the patient suffers from skin allergies, ulcers, or edema, and where large blood vessels are distributed, cupping should not be used. Do not administer cupping on a pregnant woman's abdomen and lumbosacral areas, and those suffering from high-heat and twitching symptoms should not be given cupping treatments. Do not apply the cups within 10 cm of the ribs.

If the cups are left for too long or if one has sensitive skin, small blisters will appear on the skin. Gauze should be disinfected and applied to the skin to prevent it from being rubbed and to allow blisters to heal naturally. If the blisters are relatively large, use a sterilized needle to release the fluid inside, then apply gentian violet syrup. Afterwards, apply sterilized gauze for one day and observe the affected skin area closely to prevent infection.

Chapter Fifteen
Gua Sha Scraping Therapy

Did you ever hear of or watch the movie entitled *Gua Sha Treatment*? It was directed by Chinese director Zheng Xiaolong in 2001. The story took place in the United States. The film mainly discusses Gua Sha scraping, a form of TCM natural therapy that causes some conflicts and contradictions, revealing the cultural differences between China and the US.

The *Yellow Emperor's Internal Canon of Medicine* mentions that stone needles may be used to treat certain skin-related illnesses, releasing toxins, especially when the toxins are hiding between skin and muscle. A well-known Chinese medicine professional, Li Xiangshou considers stone needles the earliest form of Gua Sha. In early times, this method was used mainly in the beginning of summer and in August, when it is especially hot and people may suffer from intolerance to the heat (called *zhu xia* in Chinese medicine). Many had great success in combating excess Heat and

Heat combined with Damp conditions through Gua Sha.

In the field of Chinese medicine, some methods for curing illnesses are simple and comfortable, but there are also recovery methods that are complicated and painful. Although simple and effective treatments are our goal, sometimes we have to suffer a bit before we can heal. Different individuals have different sensitivities to the same therapy. It is a very simple and comfortable treatment for people who like Gua Sha and acupuncture, but some people may find it painful, inducing anxiety. Choosing the method you like and can accept is important when using natural healing.

I once had the experience of using Gua Sha therapy to treat my cervical pain. At that time, the Gua Sha therapist applied forceful scraping to my neck and back for 10 minutes, but few scraping marks appeared on my skin. However, my headache and neck pain had eased. Usually I like to use jade to lightly scrape my face and scalp. Compared with facial massage, jade cools the facial skin and has a smoothing and nourishing effect, making it worth a try.

What Is Gua Sha Therapy and Its Function

Gua Sha is an ancient Chinese therapy that uses a tool to rub or scrape the skin's meridians with long strokes. Gua Sha is not a licensed practice, unlike acupuncture or moxibustion. The rate of private use of this method is much higher. In rural areas, people with less access to hospitals used whatever they had to apply this remedy at home. For example, a copper teaspoon, jade, or stones can be used to scrape the affected areas. But first, it is important to add oil/ointment on the affected area, then continue scraping with 30 to 50 strokes. Once color or *sha* (spots) appear, the symptoms will usually be alleviated.

This type of therapy can be used on areas of the body such as the back, arms, legs, and buttocks, or on the face and scalp. The force you apply should be different for different areas of the body. It also requires that the receiver have a strong constitution. People with weaker constitutions are advised to start with cupping and moxibustion.

Gua Sha can help people to deal with summer flu, fullness/heaviness in the chest, dizziness in the head, nausea, vomiting, and overall heaviness and lethargy, or joint problems and muscle issues.

Stone scraping is also applied to
certain tender points (pain points).

The purpose of Gua
Sha therapy is to help with
metabolism and local micro
blood circulation. Gentle
scraping in lymph areas is to
boost lymphatic circulation.
Gua Sha is used to help release

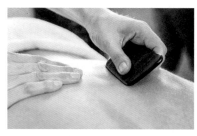

Gua Sha scraping.

whatever is congested or stagnated in the body. TCM believes that
Gua Sha, like many natural healing methods, can help expel Wind
and remove blood stagnation and reduce Heat and Dampness.

Gua Sha Theory and Mechanism

Like acupuncture, moxibustion, and cupping, Gua Sha is based on
the meridian theory, but it is more focused on meridian lines than
acupoints. The focus is sometimes a few meridian lines rather than
one. Gua Sha offers physical and chemical stimulation to the body.
The physical stimulation is the pressure and strength of the friction.
The chemical reaction comes from the oil that you use, for example
olive oil or baby oil.

Usually, the scraping is performed 30 to 50 times or more in a
downward direction. As long as you apply enough pressure, affecting
deep tissue and opening small blood vessels, some color will appear,
which is referred to as *sha*. If there is color, some people may feel a
major improvement in their bodies. Sometimes headaches, stiffness
in the neck, and other aches can be alleviated.

In Shanghai, a famous doctor by the name of Li Xiangshou,
who is well known for Gua Sha, said that Gua Sha is based on
the meridian theory, so when applying the treatment, we need to
identify the person's type first, noting, for instance, whether the
client is in an excess or weak condition. His technique includes using
more of the middle line, front, and back, then moving towards the
sides from the middle. In the limbs, he focuses more on the parts
below the elbow and below the knee. He will do deeper acupressure
on some pressure points first, then do Gua Sha combined with other
techniques such as flicking to get better results. Dr. Li's principle is
to combine all the useful natural healing methods.

The *sha* or congestion is one of Gua Sha's reaction. In medium to severe cases, it causes some micro blood veins to be broken, causing light bleeding, which is the function of the self-adjusting blood texture in one's own body. This is why Dr. Li calls Gua Sha a "therapy for stimulating potential."

Applications of Gua Sha

Based on different body conditions, one can choose different methods. But there are several principles that should be followed.

1. Choosing Materials for the Gua Sha Board

Jade is a material that is cooling and smooth, making it especially useful for facial scraping. There are also jade facial rollers that are common today, which can help blood circulation and remove Heat from the face to reduce saggy eyelids or cheek muscles.

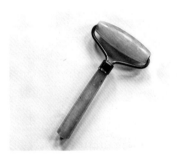

Jade facial rollers.

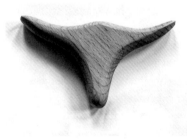

Wooden scraping board.

Gentle movements encourage more blood circulation.

Compared to other metals, copper is characterized as being highly conductive of electricity and heat. It is very durable and can be used for long periods. It is also resistant to high acidity, seawater, and alkalinity. Copper can increase the body temperature and movement of Qi. Some Doctors choose copper when treating patients. The material can also limit bacteria and microorganisms.

Wood is another option. It is friendly to the skin, has a natural aroma, and is easy to find, but it must be with rounded corners and smooth.

2. Choosing Scraping Oil

The first type is a liquid, including vegetable oil or medical oil. Vegetable oils include tea tree seed oil, olive oil, and essential oils. Medical oils include saffron oil, anti-rheumatism oil. Both can be moisturizing and nourishing for the skin, helping the pores to open to regulate blood circulation and smooth movements of Qi. This can also protect the skin during the process of scraping.

The second type is cream. You can choose very smooth textures like Vaseline or skin moisturizers or any kind of ointment with extract from motherwort.

3. Gua Sha Location and Order

After choosing the Gua Sha board and scraping oil or cream, we can start Gua Sha. Generally speaking, we start from the area of discomfort or the Ashi point (trigger point). When you feel blocked, you may try stretching. If that is not enough, you can choose Tuina massage or cupping to further release the stagnation from your body. If this is still not effective enough, you may try combining these with acupuncture or Gua Sha.

If Gua Sha is chosen for treating sunstroke (the symptoms are hotness, dizziness, mild nausea, and stiffness in the upper back or joints), we choose the upper or middle back to start with. The back is where the Governing Vessel lies, along the middle line of the back where Yang energy comes from. The general order is to go from top to bottom, or from middle outward, not back and forth. At the same time, the patient should drink cold liquids. Use the sharp part of the Gua Sha board to prick the Shuigou (GV 26) and Shixuan (EX-UE 11) points if there is dizziness or profuse sweating. Scrape along the meridian of the large intestine, especially the Quchi (LI 11) and Hegu (LI 4) points, 30 times.

Generally speaking, when doing Gua Sha, we always start with the Yang meridian, and we should only scrape in single direction. You can scrape until the skin turns a deeper red color, roughly 30 times, then it is enough. If after 30 scrapes your body is aching but there is not much color, you may stop and wait a while before trying two more times to see whether you are suitable for Gua Sha, which you will know by whether or not color appears. There are people who have stagnation, but little *sha* appears, which is fine. The key is that the symptoms are reduced.

With headaches or stiff neck, we start from the upper neck. The Governing Vessel and Gallbladder Meridians are there. Scrape along the meridians from top to bottom, inside to outside, repeating the move 30 to 50 times to help treat the symptoms. Remember that the direction for Gua Sha is always from top to bottom, neck to shoulders, or from neck all the way to the back, not the opposite directions.

If we treat the common cold and flu, we start from the area behind the neck, going from inside to outside. It must be done all in one direction, from the side of the neck all the way to the shoulder, and then to the shoulder blade. This is where the Bladder Meridian lies. After 30 movements, the treatment is complete.

During the process, if you feel more pain and discomfort or even shivering, it is better to stop. The treatment may be too strong for certain people. It is recommended that it be done step by step, with gradual increases.

4. The Angle, Strength, and Frequency of Scraping

The way in which you hold the Gua Sha board matters as well. You can hold it at a 90-degree angle. Holding it at 25 to 45 degree angle can reduce the force of the scraping. Generally speaking, if you use more force and quick movements, trying to stimulate deep tissue, there will be more red dots, which is used for those with a strong constitution. If you use lower speed, less frequent movements, it is a neutral method, and there will be fewer red dots.

Holding the Gua Sha board at 25 to 45 degree angle can reduce the force of the scraping.

According to the conditions and experience with Gua Sha, in the beginning, we advise just 10 to 15 minutes to start with, applied in a gentle manner. After one or two weeks, you can repeat the process. Wait until the red color disappears to apply the treatment again. Alternatively, first do the upper back, wait 1 to 2 days, then do the middle and lower back. This approach will require professional judgment.

Gua Sha is not suitable for everyone. Medical Gua Sha has a broader range of uses, so we will not go into more details on this.

Things to Consider

When doing Gua Sha, make sure you are in a warm environment and there is no breeze. If you cannot find a place without wind, then make sure that the body is not completely bare and that you are wearing adequate clothing.

In the summer, you should not do Gua Sha with an electrical fan facing the patient. This may cause the patient to catch the flu or reduce the effectiveness of the Gua Sha.

After Gua Sha, it is best to drink a glass of warm water. Bodily liquids need to be replenished. You can also soak the feet in hot water at the same time. Also, remember to keep the body warm after the procedure. Wait at least three hours to one day after Gua Sha before showering or swimming. If you did gentle Gua Sha for less than half an hour and there are not many red dots, you may take a shower 3 hours later. If you did whole body Gua Sha for around 2 hours and there are many deep red dots, it is better to wait one day before taking a shower.

When Not to Do Gua Sha

When one has serious diseases like cancer, heart disease, liver failure, or kidney failure, it is best not to do Gua Sha.

If one has blood conditions like weak platelets and easily bleeding, it is better not to do Gua Sha.

If one has skin allergies, skin ulcers, warts, wounds, or pimples, or on areas with many moles or scars, one may not be suited for this form of treatment.

After having suffered broken bones or serious injuries, it is also not advisable to do Gua Sha.

The weak and elderly, pregnant women, menstruating women, or patients with an empty stomach are not suitable for Gua Sha.

Do not practice Gua Sha around the genitals, belly button, eyes, or orifices. It is best for muscle areas and not veins.

Part Three

TCM Internal Management:
How Do Diet, Daily Lifestyle
and Breath Control Affect Us

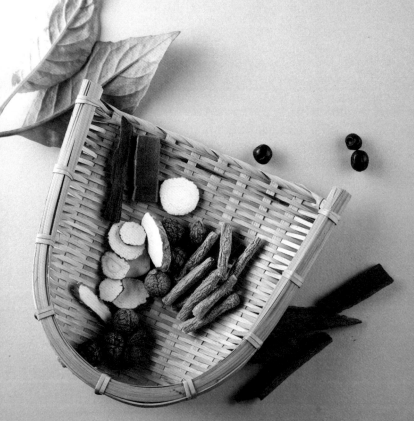

According to a 1992 survey by the World Health Organization (WHO), 40% of human health and longevity depend on genetic and objective conditions, of which 15% are genetic factors, 10% are social factors, 8% are medical conditions, and 7% are climatic conditions, while 60% depends on lifestyle and behavioral habits.

One's lifestyle and habits have a great impact on his or her health. An unhealthy lifestyle and habits are the main causes of disease. Studies show that hypertension, coronary heart disease, cerebral hemorrhaging, hyperlipidemia, diabetes, a fatty liver, and obesity all have high incident rates that directly correlate to lifestyle and psychological stress. To maintain health, improve our quality of life, and avoid diseases, it is important to make a full range of physical and mental adjustments through multiple methods, including foods, herbs, and meditation, among others.

Chapter Sixteen
Functional Foods and Recipes

In Chinese culture, the concept of cultivation of one's life is centered on maintaining health and achieving longevity by living in accordance with the laws of the universe and following the preventative health care methods as described in Parts Two and Three of this book. In this chapter, we will discuss dietary principles, meal plans to suit the season, and how to use and create functional foods.

The Concept of a Healthy Diet
The TCM concept of a healthy diet includes establishing a broad, balanced food base, making food easy to digest, thus ensuring that the amount of food is moderate and that the food suits the individual.

Building up a good sense of health consciousness in one's diet is the first way to attain physical, emotional, and mental wellness. In order to bring the body into a state of balance, we need to understand what to eat. It is a universal truth that changing the environment (climate and social environment) alongside our inherent nature affects our daily Yin-Yang balance. Because foods are also Yin or Yang in nature, they can be used as an effective method ensuring that the body's energies are balanced. It is said that we should "let food be our medicine, rather than letting the medicine be our food."

What Are Functional Foods and Drinks

Functional foods and drinks are those that play a role in health promotion and treatment or prevention of disease. Functional food was discovered in China long ago.

In ancient times, there was a rich landowner known as Mr. Qian. He was fifty years old and did not have any sons. Mr. Qian had married three wives, and eventually he had a son at the age of 53. Because of his advanced years, his family was very joyful, and they named his son Qian Fulu.

Unfortunately, due to a congenital deficiency, which was compounded by his indulgent parents, little Fulu grew up as a thin, small child. He often came down with a fever or cough, and was even too frail to stand in a gust of wind. At the age of 10, he still looked like a child of four to five.

Mr. Qian searched for experienced doctors everywhere, and his son Fulu tried almost every named remedy, but his body remained weak. A distant relative, Mrs. Wang, heard about the situation and said to Mr. Qian, "If the young master wants to strengthen his body, he should eat longan fruit."

Confused, Mr. Qian asked her, "Why, ma'am?"

Mrs. Wang explained, "When the mythical figure Nezha defeated the third prince of the Sea Dragon King to death, he dug out the prince's eyes. During that period, there was a poor child named Haizi, who was weak because of lack of nutrition, often falling sick for several months at a time. When Nezha heard about this, he asked Haizi to eat longan (dragon eye). After eating longan, Haizi recovered from his illness and became healthy, growing into a strong man. After he got married, he gave birth to 13 children, and he lived to be a hundred. After Haizi passed away, a tree grew on top of his graveyard. The tree was full of longan-like fruits. People started calling it the longan tree. Soon after, people living by the East China Sea heard of the tree, and they went to pick the longan, taking the seeds home and planting longan trees everywhere. Since then, many ate the fruit, and they all became strong and healthy."

After listening to the fairytale, Mr. Qian was pleasantly surprised. He immediately dispatched people to pick longan along the coast of the East China Sea, and the farmers dried fresh longan fruit and prepared stewed longan for Fulu to eat from time to time. Mr. Qian also instructed the farmers to grow many longan trees around the house. Since Fulu frequently ate longan, he became physically strong, which had a great impact into his adulthood.

Match Your Constitution and the Season with Appropriate Healthy Foods

It is important to match your diet to the season. In the broadest terms, this involves eating Yang foods to warm and energize the body during the winter, then eating calming Yin foods to cool the body and reduce Heat in the summer.

Similarly, it is important to ensure that your diet is aligned with your personal nature. People with a Yang constitution are usually by nature more active and forceful. They do not tolerate heat well, so in the warmer summer months, they must eat more Yin foods and reduce their intake of hot or spicy foods. The gentler nature of these Yin foods will bring one's Yang nature into balance. By contrast, those with a Yin constitution are often quieter and less energetic. They have a low tolerance for cold, so should consume more Yang foods, which are Warm or Hot, and should add spice to boost their energy.

Below are two meal plans. The first is a summer diet for a person whose constitution is naturally more Yang. The second plan presented is a winter diet for someone whose constitution is more Yin.

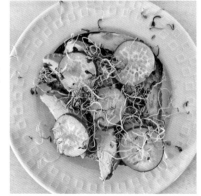

1. Summer Meal
Breakfast: avocado toast
Ingredients: 1 slice of toasted bread, 1/2 avocado, 1 red radish, salt, sprouts

Avocado toast.

Preparation: toast the bread, add avocado and radish slices and sprinkle with spouts and a pinch of salt.

Lunch: green salad

Ingredients:100 grams of grilled meat of your choice (salmon may be used), 1 cup of kale, 1 cup of spinach, 1 cup of arugula, 2 tbsp of toasted pumpkin and sunflower seeds, 1 tbsp of dry cranberries, 1/2 lemon, extra virgin olive oil, salt

Preparation: cut all the greens, prepare the condiment by mixing lemon juice, salt and oil, then mix together and place on top of the sliced meat.

Dinner: vegetarian hamburger and Mediterranean salad

Ingredients: 1 grated zucchini, 1 grated carrot, 1 pinch of curry powder, 1/2 cup of cooked rice, 1/4 cup of cooked quinoa, 1/4 cup of cooked green lentils, breadcrumbs as needed, 2 tbsp of extra virgin olive oil, mix of roasted yellow and red peppers, eggplant, and snow peas, 2 tbsp of black olives, basil, salt, pepper

Preparation: prepare the hamburgers by cooking the zucchini and carrots in a pan with some extra virgin olive oil, then add curry powder, salt. When it cools, mix with the rice,

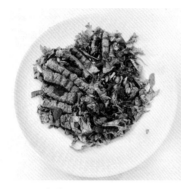

Green salad.

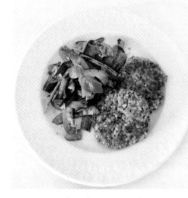

Vegetarian hamburger and Mediterranean salad.

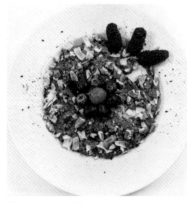

Oatmeal porridge.

quinoa, and lentils, adding breadcrumbs until the burgers reach the
desired consistency. Cook them in a pan with some olive oil. For
the Mediterranean salad, mix all the vegetables, then add the basil,
black olives, salt, and pepper.

2. Winter Day Meal

Breakfast: oatmeal porridge

Ingredients: 1/2 cup of oatmeal, 1 cup of soymilk, 1/2 cup of
blueberries, 1 piece of chocolate, 1 pinch of cinnamon, walnut,
pistachios, ground black sesame seeds, coconut flakes

Preparation: the night before, put oatmeal and soymilk in a non-
stick saucepan. In the morning, turn on the heat and cook for 15 to
20 minutes, adding liquid if it becomes sticky. Add the fresh fruits
(keep a few for garnish), cinnamon, and chocolate. Serve garnished
with crushed walnuts, pistachios, and black sesame. You can also
add goji berries, mulberries,
almond nuts, or other garnish to
taste.

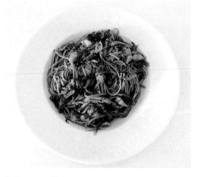

Lunch: soba noodles

Ingredients: 200 grams of
soba, 4 bok choy, 1 leek, 3 tbsp of
sesame oil, 2 tbsp of soy sauce, 1
tbsp of Chinese 5 spices (cinnamon,
star anise, Sichuan pepper, fennel
and coriander seed powder), 1 tbsp
of black sesame seeds

Preparation: cook the soba,
drain it and rinse well with cold
water. Slice the leeks and bok
choy, not too thin and sauté in
a wok for 5 minutes with the
mixture of oil and soy sauce, then
add the 5 spices. Make sure the
leaves remain crispy. Add the
soba (left slightly moist) and stir-
fry for another 5 minutes. Serve
the warm soba and sprinkle with
black sesame.

Soba noodles.

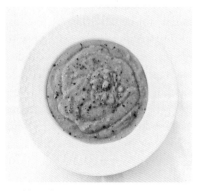

Dinner: red lentil soup

Red lentil soup.

Ingredients: 1 cup of red lentils, 2 carrots, 1 shallot, 1/2 cup of oatmeal, 1 tbsp of oil, vegetable stock, white pepper

Preparation: slice the shallots and stew with oil and a pinch of salt in a heavy-bottomed pot. Add the well-rinsed lentils and chopped carrots. Cover with vegetable stock and add the oatmeal. Cook for at least an hour, adding broth to prevent drying. Blend until soupy with a soft, dense consistency. Serve with a sprinkling of white pepper.

Suitable foods are recommended according to age, gender, and general health. The scheduling of one's food intake is another area that deserves attention, alongside the use of appropriate ingredients. There are many details surrounding the frequency of meals, the amount of each item to include in a meal, and the balance between foods based on their digestibility. Once we reach middle age, we may start to realize that skipping breakfast or eating too fast affects our physical and mental condition throughout the day. Generally, breakfast should be rich in variety and nutritious, as the entire day's store of Yang energy and one's mental energy is dependent on the various nutrients absorbed in the morning. Lunch should also include sufficient nutritious food, since it maintains our energy in the afternoon and evening. Dinner may be simple, since eating foods that are hard to digest or overeating can affect sleep. If the evening is the only time you can set aside for a solid meal, or if you have an occasional family gathering in the evening, try to avoid eating too late or taking too long to eat. For weight loss or maintenance, dinner should include no more than 20% of your daily calorie intake, with 80% being consumed for breakfast or lunch. The same is true for drinks, with 80% consumed before dinner, as this plays an important role in helping with blood and lymph circulation and excretion of waste. From a clinical perspective, physical symptoms such as flagging energy, dizziness, lower back pain, menstrual disorders, memory loss, or frequent colds will lead a TCM doctor to ask whether the patient takes breakfast every day and what they eat for breakfast. Many patients who complain of a lack of energy report that they are eating healthily, watching their nutritional intake, and exercising, but for some reason still have low energy levels. After some consultation, I often learn that these patients only eat fruit for breakfast, if they eat at all. Adjusting the diet to include a fully nutritious breakfast that includes whole grains, vegetables or fruits, and high-grade protein greatly improves their energy levels.

For the previous year, one of my patients, Ms. Wen, had only been eating a banana for breakfast, followed by a lunch of a vegetable salad and room-temperature water. During the winter, her tolerance to the cold was low, she lacked energy, and her efficiency at work declined. Eventually, she developed a menstrual disorder. Bananas and salads are by nature Cool foods, and with so little variety in her breakfast and lunch, she was not getting enough nutrition. I recommended that she add Warm cereal and a moderate amount of nuts to her breakfast regimen, then add a moderate amount of cooked beans and rhizomes to her salad for lunch. After more than a month of this altered diet, she became more energetic. Three months later, her menstrual cycle was restored to a healthy pattern.

Top Six Super Foods for Mental and Physical Energy and Longevity

This section covers important characteristics of functional foods, as identified by TCM. This includes details about the properties, tastes, channels of entry, composition, pharmacology, culinary usage, and medical applications of the six most celebrated super foods in Chinese medicine. These foods are vital to increase inner harmony between organs, strengthen the spirit, and lift the constitution.

1. Longan (Dragon Eye) 龙眼肉

Scientific name and origin: the longan is from the Sapindaceae family. Its Latin name is Euphoria longan (Lour.) Steud. In China, longans are mainly grown in Guangdong, Fujian, and Taiwan.

Properties and taste: Warm, Sweet.

Channels of entry: heart, spleen

Composition and pharmacology: longan is full of vitamins A, B, and C, glucose, and sucrose. It is a functional food that supports weight gain, improves the immune system, and has anti-bacterial, anti-

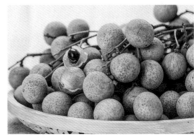
Longan (dragon eye).

cancer, and anti-hormonal functions.

Culinary usage and medical applications:

• Nourish the heart and invigorate the spleen: longan fruit strengthens weak heart Blood and spleen Qi, characterized by a yellowy face, dizziness, shortness of breath, and weariness.

• Nourish Blood to calm the mind: the longan can stimulate production of blood and improve the mood. It works against anxiety and preoccupations that affect the heart and spleen, including such symptoms as palpitations, insomnia, forgetfulness, and a poor appetite.

How to eat:

• Stew: in water, slowly stew 10 to 15 g of longan (for large dosages, no more than 60 g), along with other sliced Chinese herbs.

• Porridge: remove the skin and pit of 10 g of longan fruit and put in a pot with 100 g of rice (washed thoroughly) and 5 pitted jujubes (Chinese dates), along with sugar to taste. Add adequate water and boil into porridge. Eat once per day to relieve palpitations caused by heart Blood deficiency.

• Tea: wash 10 g of longan fruit, add to boiling water with 3 g of rock sugar. Let it steep for a while and then drink. Can be used for treating insomnia, palpitations, and excessive dreams, symptoms that demonstrate the need to strengthen the heart and spleen, and to nourish Qi and Blood.

• Jelly: using low heat, boil 1,000 g of mulberries, 500 g of longan, and sufficient water into an herb jelly. Take twice per day, 10 g per dose. This jelly benefits the liver and spleen, nourishes Blood, and brightens the eyes.

• Steam: use 20 ml of water and 50 g of dried longan and steam for 20 minutes. Eat 10 g per day for 5 days to treat Blood deficiencies.

Contraindication: people who have blockages in their middle digestive system caused by Dampness or water retention should be wary of longan. Similarly, people who have too much Heat in the heart or lung should take with caution.

2. Walnut 核桃肉

Scientific name and origin: walnuts are kernels of Juglandaceae. Latin name is Juglans regia L. Walnuts are grown in all provinces in China.

Properties and taste: Warm, Sweet

Channels of entry: kidney, lung, large intestine

Composition and pharmacology: walnuts contain fatty acids, including linoleic acid and linolenic acid. Their omega-3 fatty acids promote bone health. Preliminary research shows that walnuts can also treat coughs. They contain high levels of the amino acid L-arginine I, which is an important agent in controlling high blood pressure. An anti-oxidant called ellagic acid is present in walnuts, which may block the processes that lead to cancer.

Culinary usage and medical applications:

• Strengthen the kidney and warm the lung: as medicine, walnuts are used for asthma and coughs, including chronic cough, wheezing with shortness of breath, clear or white watery mucus, and exercise-induced asthma. These conditions are common in people who have an aversion to Cold properties and tastes during seasonal changes, especially children and the elderly.

• Treating weakness: walnuts are good for people with weakness in the back or bladder, soreness in the knees, and problems with seminal emission or urinary incontinence.

• Relieve constipation through moistening: another function of walnuts is to nourish and moisten the large intestine to treat dry stool, especially when suffering from slow movement of the colon. Similarly, they are suggested for people who experience tightness when passing stool or who have perspiration and shortness of breath after bowel movements.

How to eat:

• Powder: after grinding 10 g (daily dosage) walnuts into

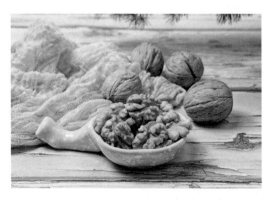

Walnuts.

powder, mix with either rice wine or water daily for 2 months to treat premature whitening of hair or poor memory. To treat kidney and urinary tract stones, use 120 g whole walnuts, 120 ml of black sesame seed oil, and 120 g white sugar. Powder the walnuts and mix all of the ingredients together. Consume 20 g 3 times per day for 6 days. Women who have recently given birth but have blocked milk ducts can mix 20 g of powdered walnuts and 20 ml warm water. Split into two portions and take one portion in the morning and one portion in the afternoon for 3 days.

• Soup: bring a root vegetable and meat with the bone to a boil, then simmer for 40 minutes. Add walnuts toward the end of the cooking, just long enough to soften. Each portion should contain 3 whole walnuts.

• Porridge: mix 50 g powdered whole walnuts, 100 g rice (pre-soaked for 20 minutes), and 300 ml of water, then cook for 50 minutes. Eat for breakfast each day for 15 days to strengthen the kidney and enhance memory and mental acuity.

• Paste: crush 10 g walnuts and 10 g black sesame seeds into powder, then mix with honey to create a paste. Take this dosage daily in the morning for at least one month to treat dry hair and scalp, split ends, premature whitening of the hair, and constipation. The paste can be added to toast, pancakes, or noodles, or another dish of your choice.

• Wine: to treat lower back pain, especially linked with cold and damp weather, soak 9 g whole walnuts in 50 ml rice wine, then steam for 10 minutes. Drink the rice wine and eat the walnuts once a day for 5 days. For the weak and elderly, add 3 g Chinese white ginseng to the recipe to steam together. Note: people suffering from stomach ulcers should not drink rice wine. Instead, make a tea of 9 g whole walnuts, 3 g white ginseng, and 75 ml water. Brew for 10 minutes, then drink the tea and eat the walnuts and ginseng.

Contraindication: those suffering from diarrhea are advised not to eat walnuts.

3. Pu'er Tea 普洱茶

Pu'er (Pu-erh) was originally produced in China's Yunnan Province, in the Xishuangbanna, Lincang, and Pu'er areas. Its harvest and preparation is very complicated. There are big, medium, and small leaves, but only the big leaves are used in the preparation

of the tea. You can buy loose
Pu'er tea in a can or compact
leaves in patty form. Storage is
very specific. The leaves should
not be kept in the kitchen as
odors may contaminate them.
They also must not be stored
under direct sunlight or in humid
conditions. Pu'er tea that is aged

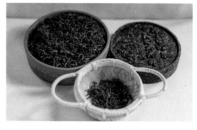

Pu'er tea.

for a longer period of time is known to have a richer taste.

Scientific name and origin: Pu'er tea is made from tender leaves
and stems of tea. Latin name is Camellia assamica (L.).

Properties and taste: raw Pu'er tea is Cold or Neutral, while
fermented or ripe Pu'er is less Cold, closer to Neutral. The taste is
Bitter and Sweet.

Channels of entry: stomach, liver, large intestine

Composition and pharmacology: the composition of Pu'er
tea is similar to that of green tea, but it contains far less reducing
sugar and tannins quantities than green tea. It also contains
pharmacologically reducing components, P-I and P-II, but the
structure is unknown. Pu'er tea extract has stronger antioxidant
effects than green tea. The two chemicals catechin and catechol
are higher in Pu'er than in other teas, which serve as great anti-
aging elements and help improve skin condition. The reducing
components P-I and P-II not only inhibit spontaneous oxidation of
linoleic acid, but also inhibit mitochondrial and microsomal reduced
coenzyme II (NADPH)-dependent lipid peroxidation in rat's liver
in experiments. Pu'er tea has anti-cancer and anti-aging properties,
and has a lipid-lowering effect. Pu'er tea extract was given to rats
on a high-cholesterol diet for 8 to 16 weeks. Plasma cholesterol
esters, triacylglycerol levels, and abdominal fat tissue contents were
lower than those in the control group. The activity of lipoprotein
lipase in abdominal adipose tissue showed a downward trend, while
adrenaline-induced lipolysis was enhanced, indicating that Pu'er tea
can promote the triacylglycerol degradation in adipose tissue.

Culinary usage and medical applications:

• Help digestion: takes care of digestive health, especially
for people with weight issues or difficulty with digesting mixed

protein foods. If there is an infection in the colon, with diarrhea and abdominal pain, Pu'er tea can help with reducing the degree of pain and stop diarrhea. It can help produce the lining inside of the digestive track to protect excess acidity, which causes ulcers and bacterial imbalances that can cause infection. When people drink to excess and experience a hangover or liver discomfort, Pu'er tea can help reduce the symptoms and eliminate liver toxins. It can also help improve indigestion, heavy bloating, and bad breath. Using it as a mouthwash can eliminate bleeding and soreness of the teeth and gums.

• Movement of Qi and expel mucous and Phlegm: Pu'er tea can help the movement of Qi, especially in the lung and spleen. Continuous long-term drinking of the tea can reduce blood lipids and blood cholesterol, helping stabilize blood pressure and prevent artery hardening.

• Cool Heat and nourish Body Fluids: expel Summer-Heat, quench thirst, treat constipation, facial pimples, and bad breath.

How to drink:

• Tea: for one person, take 5 to 10 grams of Pu'er tea and add boiling water to a porcelain pot or cup (or clay pot), stir and mix well for 30 seconds (raw) to 60 seconds (fermented), then discard the water. Add more boiling water, wait 20 seconds (raw) to 30 seconds (fermented), then discard the water (fermented Pu'er tea may need washing a third time). Finally, pour boiling water and drink. Drink 30 minutes after eating food or in the middle of the day, but never drink on an empty stomach. The best temperature is 100 degrees for fermented and 90 to 95 degrees for raw. When first drinking, you can take tea that is lighter in color and taste and not too concentrated to help you become accustomed to its taste more gradually. When drinking, it is best to first hold it under your mouth, which helps produce more saliva. Also, remember to drink Pu'er tea when it is freshly made, not after 4 to 5 hours or overnight. You can add chrysanthemum and goji berries to regulate liver function.

• Filling: like green tea, Pu'er sometimes can be combined with flowers or berries to make fillings for moon cakes or tea cakes.

• Pu'er paste: use boiled water to solute 1.5 to 3 g of Pu'er paste, then drink slowly to relieve a hangover, aid digestion, expel

Phlegm, cool stomach Heat, and produce Body Fluid. Apply 1.5 to 2 g Pu'er paste in the mouth, swallow slowly, or hold overnight to help mouth ulcers and sore throats. Topical use of Pu'er paste as a cream can relieve sunburn.

Contraindication: do not drink tea if you are experiencing depression. If you are full and gassy or are constipated or sensitive to fermented foods, you should avoid Pu'er. Otherwise, Pu'er tea is suitable for most people.

4. Sea Buckthorn 沙棘

Scientific name and origin: sea buckthorn is the mature fruit of Elaeagnaceae. Latin name is Hippophae Rhamnoides L. Originally grown in north and northwest China and in Sichuan Province.

Properties and taste: Warm, Sour, Astringent

Channels of entry: lung, stomach, liver

Composition and pharmacology: sea buckthorn contains flavonoids, including isorhamnetin, isorhamnetin-3-O-B-D-glucoside, and quercetin. It also contains fatty acid, SOD, multi-vitamins and minerals, and is super high in vitamin C. Scientific research shows that sea buckthorn improves the immune system. It controls irregular heartbeat, fights myocardial ischemia, and improves heart function. Sea buckthorn can promote hematopoietic cells and stop bleeding. It has anti-radiation, anti-oxidant, and anti-tumor properties, and also protects and treats problems in the liver.

Culinary usage and medical applications:

• Stop and eliminate phlegmatic coughs, resolve the mucus, treat bronchitis and lung abscess, and limit shortness of breath and sore throat.

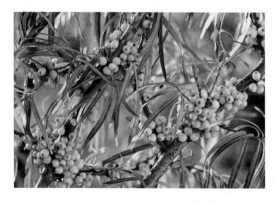

Sea buckthorn.

• Strengthen the stomach and helping digestion: treat indigestion, gastric ulcers, and enteritis. Fight symptoms including stomach pain, abdominal bloating, acid reflux, and burping with indigested food.

• Regulate blood circulation and expel stasis: treat acute injury with bruises and swelling. Help irregular menstruation and amenorrhea, reduce bruise, and regulate pigmentation.

• Topical applications usage: sea buckthorn oil agent is for skin burns, can also treat radiation damaged skin.

How to eat:

• Fresh juice: fresh sea buckthorn 50 g, drink as juice (add honey and warm water) for 3 days to treat acute sore throat.

• Oil: oral sea buckthorn oil, 10 ml twice a day for 2 to 3 months shows significant improvement in reducing pigmentation.

• Dry powder: sea buckthorn 10 g, white raisin 10 g, licorice roots 10 g to be powdered together, 2 to 3 g twice a day for 5 days for productive coughs.

• Tea: dried sea buckthorn 3 to 9 g, drink as tea for 5 days to help indigestion, frequent bruising, acid reflux, and stomach pain.

• Original pulp: buy bottled original pulp, drink 5 ml a day for maintaining good function of lung and liver systems.

• Paste: dried sea buckthorn 750 g, crush into small pieces and add 2 liters of water, cook for one hour, filtrate the solid, steam out the liquid, make the rest into a paste (like making fruit jelly), which treats stomach pain, indigestion and vitamin deficiencies.

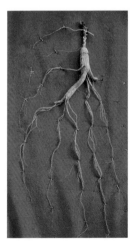

Contraindication: do not eat sea buckthorn if you are allergic to it.

5. Chinese White Ginseng 人参

Scientific name and origin: Chinese white ginseng is the root of the Araliaceae family. Latin name is Panax ginseng C.A. Mey. It is mainly grown in Jilin, Liaoning, and Heilongjiang provinces of China. Cultivated, it is called *yuan shen* (garden ginseng), and in the wild, it is called *shan shen* (mountain ginseng).

Chinese white ginseng.

Properties and taste: slightly Warm,

Sweet, slightly Bitter

Channels of entry: lung, spleen, heart, kidney

Composition and pharmacology: the root contains various ginsenosides, such as ginsenosides Ra1, Ra2, Rb2, Rb3, Rc, Rd, Re, Rf, Ro; Rg1, Rg2, and Rh1. Chinese white ginseng has a two-way regulation for sedation and excitement of the central nervous system. It can enhance the non-specific immunity of the body. It regulates blood pressure in two ways, with a similar effect as cardiac glycosides. It can indirectly promote the adrenal cortex function and has an anti-diuretic effect. It increases the erythropoietin content in the marrow, liver, and spleen, and it reduces blood sugar and has anti-inflammatory and anti-tumor properties.

Culinary usage and medical applications:

• Strengthen Original Qi: for people with serious Qi deficiencies, as when someone has lost a good deal of blood or liquid from vomiting or diarrhea and are severely dehydrated. Symptoms include cold perspiration with a weak pulse. Sometimes it is used on its own. Using only 10 to 30 grams ginseng, one can make a soup, or if there are ready-made forms of a concentrated paste or tincture, these can be used to strengthen Qi.

• Strengthen spleen Qi deficiency: indicated by mental and physical fatigue, poor appetite, fullness and bloating in the upper abdominal area, or vomit or diarrhea, among other symptoms. Ginseng can be combined with cooked licorice and poria cocos to combat these symptoms.

• Strengthen lung Qi deficiency: if experiencing shortness of breath, lack of activity, lethargy, or spontaneous sweating, ginseng can be consumed with walnuts.

• Strengthen Qi and nourish Body Fluids: can be used for the rehabilitation and recovery after acute illness. Symptoms include thirst and excessive perspiration. Some people even feel dryness in the orifices, such as nose and eyes. It can also be applied to chronic conditions, such as Qi and Yin deficiencies and diabetes, especially when there are symptoms of thirst, spontaneous sweating, and frequent urination.

• Regenerate Blood, calm the mind, and increase mental capacity: symptoms include forgetfulness or lack of concentration, sometimes combined with dream-disturbed sleep, a pale face, and dizziness or weakness. Ginseng can be combined with longan fruit and angelica root.

How to eat:

• Steamed: you can use ginseng to make tea, steaming instead of boiling, using 5 to 10 g cut into very small pieces. Add 50 ml of mineral water and soak the ginseng overnight, then steam for one hour and drink a small quantity each day for 5 to 7 days. You should reheat it each time you drink. You may eat the cooked ginseng as well.

• Soup: you can combine ginseng with chicken to make a soup, using just 10 g of ginseng. If you have never eaten it before, you may start off with smaller quantities.

• Steeping: make tea by steeping slices of ginseng or mixing ginseng powder with boiling water.

• You can also ingest ginseng capsules, tincture, abstracts, or paste, then take an corresponding dosage, for example 1 g each day.

• Decoction: treat recurrent mouth ulcers by boiling 20 to 30 g (2 weeks supply) ginseng into a decoction. Drink 30 to 50 ml before breakfast and eat a few pieces of cooked ginseng each day for a week. Subsequently, you may drink the decoction 2 to 3 times a week. Your ulcers will show great improvement after 3 to 6 months.

Contraindication:

People with excess or Heat syndromes should not use ginseng.

When taking ginseng, you should avoid drinking tea and coffee and avoid eating radishes and grapes. These will interfere with the body's absorption of the ginseng.

When preparing ginseng, do not use steel or metal utensils or pots. The best material is porcelain.

6. Fiveleaf Gynostemma Herb 绞股蓝

Scientific name and origin: the whole herb of the Cucurbitaceae family. Latin name is Gynostemma pentaphyllum (Thunb) Makino. It grows mainly in Shaanxi Province, south of

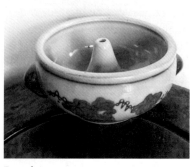
Porcelain pot.

the Qinling Mountains and the
Yangtze River, and in Yunnan,
Hubei, and Hunan provinces in
China, and parts of India, Nepal,
and Sikkim.

Properties and taste: Cool,
Bitter, slightly Sweet

Channels of entry: lung,
spleen, kidney

Composition and

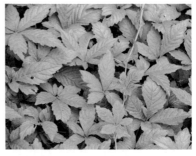

Fiveleaf gynostemma herb.

pharmacology: fiveleaf gynostemma herb contains high gypenosides,
gynostemma polysaccharides, flavonoids, terpenoids, saponins,
and sugar. Their effects include prevention of tumors, increased
longevity, and controlling blood cholesterol and hypoglycemic
activity. It protects the liver and improves immunity as well. Modern
research shows it can also prevent ulcers, tranquillize and encourage
better sleep, and relieve pain.

Culinary usage and medical applications: fiveleaf gynostemma
herb grown in the south has a relatively high medicinal content. It
is called "southern ginseng," or by the colloquial name "longevity
herb." The Qinba mountain area of Shaanxi Province was identified
as the global gypenosides gold producing area and is known as the
"fiveleaf gynostemma herb valley."

• Strengthen Qi and nourish Yin for both Qi and Yin
deficiencies, with symptoms being fatigue and lethargy, shortness of
breath, dry mouth, and thirst.

• Tone lungs and moisten Dryness, effective for lung
deficiencies, combined with a Heat deficiency, usually for chronic
cough with no mucus or coughing for long periods with yellow
sticky mucus. It has also been used to help treat lung cancer, with
a dose of 15 to 30 grams each day. Clean the fiveleaf gynostemma
herb thoroughly, then cut into small pieces. Put it into a pot with
500 ml of mineral water and cook for 30 minutes. Pour the liquid
out and repeat again with 300 ml of mineral water. Mix these two
cooked liquids together and add 30 ml of honey for taste. TCM
teaches that cooking the ingredient at least twice ensures that you
are getting the most benefit from it. Finish this quantity in the
course of one day.

• Nourish the heart and calm the mind for both spleen and heart deficiencies. It can help with paleness, fullness in the chest, palpitations, and even dull pain in the chest, as well as asthmatic breathing after little exercise and a weak or irregular pulse.

• Tone kidney and consolidate kidney Essence. Symptoms include weakness in the lower back and knees, irregular menstruation, involuntary semen emissions, and nocturnal emissions.

How to eat:

• Making a tea: use 15 grams that have been cleansed thoroughly, cook with boiling water for 15 minutes, then continue using the ingredient by boiling it with more water for 5 minutes at a time until there is no more flavor. This is often used for people with diabetes. Add honey or dates to make the taste more palatable.

• Making a soup: use 15 grams of the herb and 8 pieces of dried longan. Bring them to a boil and simmer for 20 minutes. Eat the longan and drink the soup. This will help with focus and concentration and will also foster better sleep.

• Ingesting tablets and capsules: take 3 grams 3 times a day to help regulate blood lipids. Tea bag forms are also available at the pharmacy.

• Gynostemma pentaphyllum extract: gypenosides tabellae (绞股蓝总甙片) to treat the early stages of diabetic nephropathy.

Contraindication:

• Deficiency and Cold syndrome

• People with diarrhea and stomach aversions to cold food

Chapter Seventeen
The Chinese Materia Medica and Prescriptions

Plants are the bond that connects humans and nature. The plants we have access to are divided into two categories, foods and herbs. Plants that are used as food are further divided into three major categories according to their functions and features. The first is elementary healthy food that helps our body maintain itself on a daily basis. The second is food for pleasure, relaxing, and socializing as a means to satisfy certain emotional needs (in moderation, of course). The last is for the purpose of healing, reducing risks of

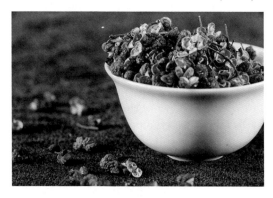

Sichuan pepper.

illness, and maintaining and promoting good health. These three categories, if kept safe and clean, can be applied to most people at any time, except for those who have an intolerance or allergies.

Herbs are divided into three grades according to their side effects, namely top grade, middle grade, and low grade. Foods with healing effects and herbs in the top grade refer to the same group of plants. We refer to them as having "dual-use for Chinese materia medica and food" (about 110 kinds of Chinese medicine are also used as foods, such as cinnamon and Sichuan pepper).

Traditional Chinese medicine is often referred to as herbal medicine. It is a discipline that studies the theories and clinical application of herbs, which is one of the fundamental disciplines of all areas of TCM. The classes and syllabus' of Chinese medical universities vary in their focal points due to the differences among the specializations offered. If a student majoring in TCM plans to become a pharmacist after graduation, they will have to focus on learning about the location, collection, origins, process, and distinguishing of herbs. If the student plans to become a TCM doctor, they will have to focus more on learning about the nature and healing mechanism of the herbs, as well as the formula, doses, and taboos associated with certain types.

The Concept of the Chinese Materia Medica
The Chinese materia medica is also called the Han materia medica. It originated from the ancient Han ethnic group and was developed by ancient Han scholars. Its fundamental theories were formed in ancient times by the Han ethnic group, forming an integral part of the Han

ethnic cultural system. The Han materia medica is herbal-based medicine. The idea "herbal-based" comes from the conclusion of the pioneers of the practice that medicines are most abundant among the herbs, and herbs are the foundation of all medicine. Herbal medicine accounts for a large majority of all Chinese medicines, and it is widely used. Herbal medicine is a science that studies the herbs used by the Han people. It is mainly based on plants, but also covers animals and minerals. In this book, we will only discuss plants.

Origins of Chinese Herbal Medicine

There is a long-standing history of studying plants in China. There are many legends of the pioneers who tasted different herbs in the Shen Nong Age. The Shen Nong Age was approximately around the same time as the New Stone Age. People at that time had developed traditional agriculture and started to gain a sense of the nature and healing effects of different plants and natural herbs. The word "tasting" implies that the nature and healing effects of the herbs were discovered by trying them out on human bodies. Some herbs demonstrated amazing features and were even able to heal two completely opposite conditions. For example, Chinese angelica root can regulate the menstrual cycle, and treat both excessive and light menstruation. The Schisandra berry has the double effect of both increasing and decreasing blood sugar, while notoginseng has the double effect of stopping bleeding and quickening blood circulation.

The earliest Chinese herbal medical work in China is *Shen Nong's Classic of the Materia Medica*, which was completed in the Han dynasty (202 BC–AD 220). The book records 365 types of herbs and was written by different doctors over a long period of

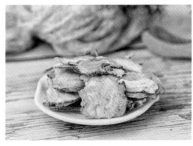

Chinese angelica root.

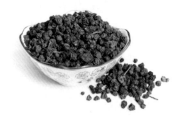

Schisandra berry.

time. There are three volumes in the book, each describing one grade of herbs. The words are simple and concise, and the book contains the essence of Chinese pharmacy practice. It was written in the "Herbal Classic, Preface" of *Shen Nong's Classic of Materia Medica* that the 120 top grade

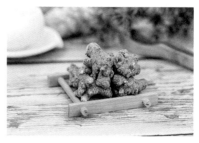

Notoginseng.

herbs are the main herbs which serve the purpose of connecting humans with the universe by strengthening, nourishing, and maintaining life energy. These herbs are non-toxic and will not harm the body, even if taken over a long period of time. They include ginseng, licorice root, rehmannia, and jujube. The 120 middle grade herbs are auxiliary herbs which serve to connect humans with their surroundings by supporting the constitution and regulating the physical state. Depending on the types, some are toxic and some are not, so it is important to distinguish their nature, such as lily bulb, Chinese angelica root, longan, and goldthread root. The 125 low grade herbs are those that are only used occasionally. They connect humans with the earth by treating diseases. They are often toxic and should not be taken for longer than necessary. These include herbs such as rhubarb root (Radix et Rhizoma Rhei), Aconitum carmichaeli Debx, and Fructus Crotonis. We can understand the maintenance of human health through the analogy of a car. There are three types of Chinese herbal medicines: ① fundamental fuel, or medicine used often to keep our body and spirit running smoothly. ② service adjustment, or medicine used for certain period or during seasonal changes as necessary. ③ overhaul, or medicine used to pull the physical condition back onto the right track when the body gives an alarming signal, like in a car. This is why many people believe in and practice Chinese herbal medicine.

In the Ming dynasty, Li Shizhen (1518–1593) compiled the *The Grand Compendium of Materia Medica*, a summative masterpiece of pharmacology in China. It consists of 52 volumes and is divided into sixteen sections and sixty categories, covering 1,892 kinds of medicine and containing more than 1,000 illustrations. The book was a great contribution to practical taxonomy and natural history.

It covers a wide range of topics and provides certain insights into biology, chemistry, astronomy, geography, geology, mining, and even history. It has had a positive impact on the spread of Chinese medicine worldwide.

The *Chinese Materia Medica* was continuously expanded and improved by generations of doctors over time. At present, there are many new books on TCM herbal medicine, such as the *Great Dictionary of Chinese Herbal Medicine*. These huge books cover a wide ranges of specialized fields. They bring herbal medicine to new heights in various aspects. The one that can best represent the accomplishments of herbal medicine is the follow up version of *Chinese Pharmacopoeia*.

Properties of Herbal Medicine

The nature and function of herbs is to regulate the four energies (Cold, Heat, Warmth, and Cool), five tastes (Sour, Bitter, Sweet, Pungent, and Salty), and their channels of entry (see details in Chapter Two to Four of Part One). Apart from these features, herbs also present the properties of ascending and descending or floating and sinking.

The four properties mean the four tendencies according to which they work within the human body.

1. Ascending

To rise, lift, or elevate. All herbs that treat pathogenesis of falling (sinking) conditions have the function of ascending. For example, Astragalus root can lift the Yang Qi and treat chronic diarrhea, ptosis, or anal and uterine prolapse.

2. Descending

To decline, drop, and suppress. All herbs that treat pathogenesis

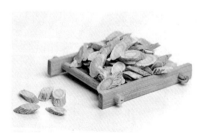

of upward inversion or rising conditions have the function of descending. For example, clove has a warm nature that dispels Coldness in the body and suppresses a rising trend. It treats vomiting and hiccups.

3. Floating

To go upwards, to lift and

Astragalus root.

bring to the surface. All herbs that treat superficial conditions or illness at the onset location have the function of evaporating. For example, peppermint can treat headaches and red eyes at the onset of a flu.

4. Sinking

To go downwards. All herbs that treat deep-rooted conditions or illnesses located on the inside have the function of sinking. For example, chive seeds can guide medicine to the lower part of the body, treating frequent urination, excessive vaginal discharge, and soreness in the waist and knees, conditions which are rooted deeper in the body.

To conclude, all evaporating herbs can lift the Qi and direct it outward, such as those for raising the Yang Qi, exterior-releasing, dispelling the Coldness, and inducing vomiting. All sinking herbs can go downward and direct the Qi inward, such as those for clearing Heat, downward-draining, promoting the movement of water, astringent, or tranquillizing coughs and hiccups.

The four trends of ascending, descending, floating, and sinking are the four different categories of the medicine and serve as the guiding principle in clinical prescription. Conditions can occur at the upper or lower part, or on the surface or inside of the human body. Different diseases are distinguished by their rising and sinking trends. The herbs should be applied according to the different locations and trends of the illness.

Channels of entry: the four trends also provide an inductive method for understanding the medicinal natures of the herbs and are closely related to the channels of entry in clinical application. For example, lung problems such as coughs should be treated with herbs that go into the Lung Meridien, but with a distinction in the trends. Coughs that are caused by exterior Coldness and result in the suppression of the lung Qi should be treated with evaporating herbs such as perilla. Chronic coughs caused by weakness of lung Qi should be treated with sinking herbs that astringe the lungs and tranquillize the cough such as schisandra berry. To treat rising conditions, sinking herbs should be applied, but it must first be made clear which meridian the herbs will enter. For example, persimmon calyx goes to the Stomach Meridian and is therefore applicable to rising stomach Qi and hiccups. Almond goes to the Lung Meridien and is therefore applicable to rising of lung Qi and asthmatic coughs.

Generally speaking, the four different trends are related to the nature and texture of the herbs. From the perspective of taste and nature, ascending and floating herbs are generally Pungent-Sweet in taste and Warm in nature, whereas descending and sinking herbs are generally Bitter, Sour, or Salty in taste and Cool in nature. From the perspective of texture, ascending and evaporating herbs are often in the form of flowers or leaves which are light, whereas descending and sinking herbs are often in the form of seeds or fruits which are heavy. However, the process or preparation of the herbs may cause changes in these trends. For example, when fried in liquor, the trend ascends. When fried with ginger, the trend disperses. When fried with vinegar, the trend astringes, and when fried in salt, the trend descends.

The Processing of Herbal Medicine

Not all natural medicine is Chinese medicine. The concept and connotation of Chinese medicine does not simply mean being natural, although most herbs are taken from nature. Some herbs can be used directly, but they are not Chinese medicine in the truest sense. Those that are called Chinese medicine, first and foremost, are those that have been processed in various ways. The processing not only clears the dust and dirt, making the medicine easier to use, but also eliminates or reduces toxic parts and their side effects and enhances the effectiveness by changing the nature of the herbs. For instance, raw rehmannia clears Heat and cools the Blood, but after being steamed with liquor and dried, it becomes Warm and is able to nourish the kidneys and the Blood.

There are different ways of processing, such as with water, fire, or the combination of water and fire. Water processing can be further classified into washing, dipping, soaking, preserving in salt, blanching, and other treatments. Fire processing can be further classified into calcining, roasting in ashes, roasting, baking, stir-frying, and similar processes. Water-and-fire

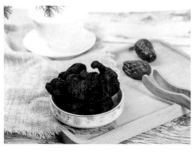

Raw rehmannia.

process can be further classified into steaming, boiling, extracting, and so forth. Each method contains multiple detailed procedures, each of which has a special purpose. Some of the processes have become closely kept secrets.

In stir-baking, the herbs are first heated in a pan, then stir-fried until they have a light yellow tint or turn completely black, depending on the requirements of the patient's condition. When fried to a light yellow color, Rhizoma Atractylodis (ovate atractylodes) will more effectively strengthen the spleen and increase the appetite. Depending on the actual needs, the effect of the herbs can be strengthened by frying with liquor, vinegar, or salt water. For example, Chinese angelica root, when fried with liquor, is more effective for quickening the blood.

Chinese medicine should not be applied by simply mixing different herbs, but rather through different formulas that are set according to the four energies and five tastes and the principle of top grade, middle grade, and low grade. According to the needs, medicine can be taken as tea, decoction, pills, powder, or paste (patches). To sum up, Chinese medicine does not simply refer to natural herbs. Neither can they be mixed or substituted for one another.

The Theory of Combination

In TCM, combination means using more than two different herbs at the same time, according to the nature of the herbs and the specific conditions of the disease. The cause and development of a disease is often complicated and is constantly changing. Often, a patient presents mixed symptoms, such as co-existence of deficient and excessive syndromes, or mixed Cold and Heat conditions. Sometimes we may even have to look at more than one disease at the same time. This makes it difficult to treat a condition with just one type of herb. Typically, more than two herbs will be used together. The interaction of the herbs will enhance or decrease their original individual effect. Sometimes it suppresses or eliminates the side effects, but it can also incur or increase the side effects. Therefore, herbs must be chosen and matched carefully according to the principles of formulation. The pioneers of TCM describe the relations among the individual herbs and the matching of herbs as six sentiments (six kinds of matches). Apart from those herbs that are used alone, the six matches point us toward proper matching and combination.

1. Single Herb

A single herb can be used without being combined with any other herbs and still be effective. For example, in ginseng soup, only ginseng is used, and it is enough to treat the critical symptoms caused by the weakness of Qi, dizziness, and blackouts after childbirth or the loss of consciousness.

2. Enhancement (Mutual Promotion between Two Herbs)

Combining herbs that have a similar nature and effect can enhance each individual herb. For example, Chinese ephedra combined with cinnamon sticks can have stronger effect in warming the body and inducing perspiration. Rhubarb root combined with natrii sulfas work better for draining Heat.

3. Support (Mutual Enhancement between Two Herbs)

The effects of one main herb can be enhanced by another supportive herb which has some similarities or which treats the same conditions even if the nature and function is not quite the same. For example, astragalus root supplements Qi and promotes water when used with poria, which also promotes water, so the effect is amplified.

4. Fear (Mutual Restraint between Two Herbs)

The toxin or side effect of one herb can be reduced or completely eliminated by the other. For example, the side effect of raw pinellia rhizome can be reduced or eliminated by ginger, which TCM describes as raw pinellia rhizome "fearing" ginger.

5. Kill (Mutual Detoxication between Two Herbs)

One herb can "kill" another herb's toxin or side effect, such as ginger "killing" pinellia rhizome's toxicity.

6. Dislike (Mutual Inhibition between Two Herbs)

One herb is less effective or becomes completely ineffective when used with another herb. For example, ginseng dislikes radish seeds, because its effect of supplementing Qi can be diminished by radish seeds.

7. Contradiction (Antagonism between Two Herbs)

When two contradicting herbs are used together, they will become poisonous or have stronger side effects. For example, veratrum nigrum (black false hellebore) cannot be used with ginseng and herbaceous peony or it may produce strong toxicity and side effects.

The application of these six sentiments can be summarized by four scenarios.

- Herbs that enhance each other's effect should be used more often, as enhancement and support.
- Herbs that may reduce the effect of other herbs should be used carefully and less often.
- Some herbs must be used if certain aggressive and poisonous herbs are used in the formula, since they can reduce the toxin and side effect.
- Some herbs must not be used together since they discount or even completely eliminate each other's effects.

Based on these principles, it can be inferred that the application of both single herbs and the combinations of different herbs are summarized and improved over a long period through the accumulation of experience. These formulas are the main form of application of Chinese medicine. A prescription consists of processed herbs that are matched by a certain philosophy and certain dosages. Prescription is the development of formulas and is an advanced form of combination.

Dosage of Herbs

The quantity of herbs used is determined according to the condition and progression of the disease, as well as the constitution, age, and build of the patient. For example, smaller dosages should be given to children and seniors, or if the symptom is superficial and mild and doesn't last long. Larger dosages are given to adults that are young and robust or if the symptom is complicated and its roots deeper in the body.

Method for Herb Use

Herbs are normally taken as decoction or applied externally. The general rule for oral herbal medicine is that the herbs are to be taken twice a day, usually drunk half an hour after a meal. Tonic herbs are to be taken before meals. Detoxifying herbs and laxatives should be taken on an empty stomach. Herbal medicine is given immediately in cases of acute or urgent illness. External applications include soaking, plasters, and herb oils.

Taboos (Contradiction)

Though medicines can cure diseases, they also have side effects which can harm the human body. For example, if herbs with a Cold nature are used excessively, they will damage the Yang Qi. If herbs that clear Heat are used excessively, they may damage the Body Fluids. If aggressive herbs are used too frequently, they may harm the Defensive Qi of the body. Too much nourishing medicine can also ruin people's appetite. During pregnancy, the improper application of herbs can lead to a miscarriage or pre-mature birth. The pioneers of TCM attached great importance to taboos during pregnancy. Herbs such as rhubarb root, peach kernels, cinnamon, and other draining and stasis-expelling herbs, as well as very Warm herbs with a Pungent taste and herbs that open the orifices and meridians should not be given to pregnant women, or should given very carefully and only when it is absolutely necessary.

Categories and Examples of Herbs According to Their Nature and Function

Exterior-releasing means using herbs to treat onset or surface illness. Surface illness are distinguished as Cold or Hot. If it is a Cold flu, we use Warm or Hot herbs, like ginger and cinnamon stick. If it is Hot flu, we use Cool or Cold herbs, like mint and chrysanthemum.

Heat-clearing means using herbs to treat an illness inside the body, with various parts of body and degrees of Heat type.

Heat-clearing and Fire-draining: lotus plumule

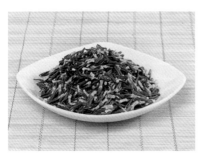

Liver-clearing and eye-brightening: cassia seed

Heat-clearing and Blood-cooling: dried or fresh rehmannia

Heat-clearing and toxin-releasing: honeysuckle, dandelion

Heat-clearing and Damp-dispelling: goldthread root

Soft heat-clearing: sweet wormwood

Lotus plumule.

Downward-draining means using herbs to treat illnesses related to constipation, with relatively strong purgatives or moistening herbs.

Downward-sinking: senna leaf, aloe vera

Downward-moisturising: honey, hemp seeds

Promoting the movement of water and percolating Dampness means using herbs to treat various parts of blockages caused by Dampness and water, such as edema caused by Dampness and water in the muscles and joints.

Dampness-removing by diuresis: poria, azuki bean, pearl barley

Dampness-transforming means using herbs to treat various parts of blockages caused by Phlegm-Dampness, for instance, Phlegm obstructing the lungs and causing coughs or asthma, or Dampness affecting the digestive system and generating fullness of the stomach and abdominal bloating. Herbs include herba eupatorii and flos magnoliae officinalis.

Wind-Damp-dispelling means using herbs to treat the meridians, muscles, tendons, and joints for ailments caused by Wind-Damp. These herbs can dispel Wind and infiltrate Dampness. For example, rheumatic stagnates the meridians and causes joint pain, tendon spasms, or skin and muscle numbness. Herbs include mulberry stick (twig), fructus chaenomelis, luffa, and cucurbitaceous plants. They have a Cool nature and Sweet taste, and they enter the Lungs, Stomach, and Liver Meridians. The function is to clear the toxins and activate the meridians, and they are suitable for soreness and pain in the ligaments, bones, and ribs, and for breast lumps. The normal dose is 5 to 15 grams, and it should be taken as decoction.

Qi-regulating means using herbs to treat the Qi's stagnation or inversion.

Tangerine pith and the film on the madrine petals has a Neutral nature and Bitter taste. The function is to transform Phlegm, regulate Qi, and smooth the meridians. It is suitable for transforming stagnating Phlegm in the meridians and can treat coughs and chest pains. The normal dose is 5 to 7 grams, and it should be taken as a soup.

Outside of tangerine peel and the fruit of Citrus reticulata Blanco has a Bitter flavor and Warm-Pungent nature. It is suitable for excessive Phlegm and coughs, as well as indigestion and

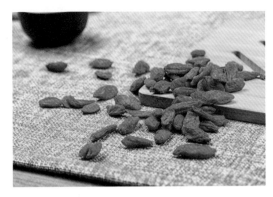

Wolfberries.

stomachaches. The normal dose is 3 to 10 grams, and it should be taken as a soup.

Blood-quickening and stasis-dispelling means using herbs to treat blood stagnation or blood stasis. Herbs include peach kernels, safflower, saffron, and turmeric.

Supplementing means using herbs to treat various weaknesses and weak functioning of the organs. TCM summarizes them as deficiency of Qi, Blood, Yin, and Yang.

Supplementing Qi: ginseng, chinese yam, licorice root

Nourishing Blood: angelica, longan fruit, mulberry

Enriching Yin: wolfberry, lily bulb, silver ear

Fortifying Yang: raspberry, walnut, chive seed

There are eight categorizations based on function that are most often employed as healing methods based on the eight contradictions. The eight contradictions are outer and inner, Cold and Heat, weak and solid, Yin and Yang. The eight methods are sweating, vomit-inducing, downward-draining, harmonizing, warming (Cold-expelling), Heat-clearing, food-dispersing, and supplementing.

Due to the development of medicine and the rising needs in clinical practice, there are actually more than eight methods employed. Given the constraints of a short volume such as this, we mainly discuss only three of the eight methods.

Sweating, also referred to as exterior releasing, is a method which induces the perspiration of the patient with a prescription of exterior-releasing herbs, so that the external factor is released and the symptoms improved. Ginger and white spring onion are examples of such herbs.

Downward-draining, also called sinking, is a method which expels the stagnation in the bowels and excessive water in the body, releasing the Dampness by inducing bowel movements with a prescription of herbs that have downward-draining functions, such as Rhubarb root (Radix et Rhizoma Rhei) or hemp seed. This method is mainly applicable to interior excess conditions, and is sometimes also used in mixed conditions of weakness and excess.

Tonic weakness supplementing, also called supplementing, is a method that removes the symptoms of weakness by using a prescription of nourishing or strengthening herbs. This method is applicable to weakness in the Qi and Blood as well as Yin and Yang in the body caused by various factors. The prescription enhances the function of the gut and nourishes the body, so that the metabolism is accelerated and immune system performance improved, allowing the body to heal quickly. Herbs include licorice root and angelica root.

Herbal health care began in the Han dynasty's Chinese pharmacy monograph *Shen Nong's Classic of the Materia Medica*, which contains 365 kinds of Chinese medicine, in which 120 top grade herbs have a nourishing effect. In terms of their efficacy, many words and statements were uttered related to such things as lightening the body and anti-age, longevity, lubricating the skin, or enhancing beauty. At the time, other books also had records of using herbs such as almond, wolfberry, poria, and polygonatum root that have healthcare functions.

Prescriptions of TCM

We have previously discussed TCM herbal medicine, its theoretical basis, and its categories. Prescription is another important branch of TCM that is closely associated with herbal medicine. The categories of herbs and prescriptions are consistent with and linked to one another. There are exterior-releasing herbs, which are used to create exterior-releasing formulas. Before prescribing an exterior-releasing formula, we need to determine how many exterior-releasing herbs we have acquired. For instance, there are pungent-warm or pungent-cool exterior-releasing herbs that we should use in order to release the Cold or Hot types of common cold. When you suffer from the onset of a Cold type of flu (chills, no sweat, itchy throat), you can relieve the symptoms with a single herb such as ginger or cinnamon in a tea, but a TCM doctor might consider using a pungent-warm exterior-releasing formula, such as a cinnamon decoction formula, which includes cinnamon sticks, white peony root, licorice root, ginger, and jujube, or a scallion and fermented soybean decoction, which includes white spring onion and black bean sauce (fermented soybean).

From this it is evident that a formula or prescription is the combination of several herbs which are used together according to the rules of TCM and its healing principles. Prescription as an academic discipline investigates the correlation between healing methods and formula constituents, the variation and rules of the formulas, and its dosage form and clinical application. In short, it is a science that studies how to improve the healing effects of herbs by finding the best combination.

Concept of Prescription

Prescribing suitable herbs in the right quantity is the next step once treatment methods have been determined through dialectical analysis. A proper prescription consists of herbs that are matched according to the principles of hierarchy and proportion. There are strict rules to be followed when prescribing a formula. The Chinese word for prescription is 方剂 (fang ji). Fang means methods and categories, and ji is equivalent to order, which describes the status when an array of objects is put together in a neat order. When they are put together, the word indicates the rules or patterns, for example in height or in quantity.

A formula is formed by certain rules and methods. When prescribing a formula, we must first choose the main herb according to the main symptom presented, then complete the formula with supporting herbs. The quantity of Warm and Cold herbs, application methods, and duration must be considered. The nature of the herbs must be suitable for the patterns (symptoms), like a key made to fit a specific lock.

Origin of Prescriptions

There have been records of using single herbs for treating diseases since China's early history. After centuries of practice and study, the early pioneers of TCM learned to combine different herbs to

make decoctions, powders, or pills. Such was the earliest shape of
prescriptions. The *Yellow Emperor's Internal Canon of Medicine*, the oldest
medical book currently available, laid the foundation for prescriptions.
It created a system for treatment methods and set rules and principles
for them. The book recorded the constituents, combinations, and
applications of thirteen types of formulas and introduced the view that
prescriptions should follow the theoretical basis of sovereign, minister,
assistant, and guide (see details of these items later in this chapter).

At the end of Eastern Han dynasty, Zhang Zhongjing made
great contributions to the art of prescription preparation in his book
Treatise on Cold Damage and Miscellaneous Diseases. Most importantly,
he established a dialectical theoretical system. Each symptom has
an underlying cause. The treating method and prescription has to
be chosen based on the causes of the ailment. That is to say, they
must merge theory, method, prescription, and herbs to make it an
integrated system in clinical practice.

Further, Dr. Zhang formulated more than 300 prescriptions that
have proved effective in practice. Contemporary practitioners refer to
these prescriptions as classical formulas.

In addition, Dr. Zhang originated many base formulas, which
drove the development of prescriptions after his time. These base
formulas reflect many fundamental principles, for example, pairing
Rhizoma Atractylodis (ovate atractylodes) with poria is suitable for
pathogenesis (symptoms) caused by weak Qi and blocked Dampness.
Dr. Zhang's use of the appropriate number of herbs in precise
dosages have also made a long-lasting impact on the development of
prescriptions in the centuries that followed. Zhang Zhongjing is still
held in high esteem as the pioneer of prescriptions.

Formulas for Universal Relief, a medical book compiled in the
Ming dynasty containing 61,739 formulas, offers more prescriptions
than any book of its kind. The highest accomplishment among
contemporary studies is the *Encyclopedia of Chinese Medicinal Formulas*.

Constituents of Formulas

Making formulas involves a process of choosing the proper herbs and
determining their dosage, form, and application according to certain
principles once the symptoms have been analyzed dialectically. The
process from creating formulas to determining their final formation

of the prescription reflects the philosophy of holism and dynamic changes. Holism refers to the alignment of humans and nature through a balanced Yin and Yang in the body and the alignment of body and mind. Healing methods are based on the principle of tracking the deep-rooted causes, adjusting Yin and Yang, complementing weakened Qi, and draining blockages. Dynamic changes include the adjustments made according to the individual, timing, and location. For example, when treating a common cold, the formula for colds caused by Cold forces is different from that for those caused by Heat. Even if the cause is the same, the formula for treating a robust young adult is different from that used for an elderly person. This is one of the differences between TCM and Western medicine. Western medicine values drugs more than herbal or natural formulas, viewing drugs as the base unit of healing. Even when there is a formula, it is reversed back into a drug. TCM, on the other hand, attaches equal importance to Chinese materia medica and formulas, perhaps placing even more emphasis on formulas.

Creating formulas is a process of matching properly chosen herbs and determining dosage according to the principle of "sovereign, minister, assistant, and guide" following a process of dialectical analysis. It is more complicated than simply putting a bunch of herbs together.

Sovereign medicinal herbs are those that meant to play the major role in treating the main disease or symptoms. According to the current needs, one or more herbs can be used.

Minister medicinal herbs are those supporting the sovereign herbs in order to enhance their effect or treat side symptoms. According to the current needs, one or more herbs can be used.

Assistant medicinal herbs are those restraining the sovereign and minister herbs in order to remove or reduce their toxicity or to adjust the flavors and help the medicine take shape. According to the current needs, one or more herbs may be used.

Guide medicinal herbs are those used as a catalyst, normally only one herb is used as guide herb.

The cinnamon stick decoction formula recorded in the *Treatise on Cold Damage* serves as an example. The decoction mainly treats common colds caused by external Coldness. Symptoms include a high body temperature, an intolerance of wind, sweating, light red color of the tongue with a white coating, and a slower pulse. The function is to release Cold energy by expelling external factors from the surface, strengthening the Defensive Qi, and regulating Nutrient Qi and Defensive Qi. The formula for the decoction is:

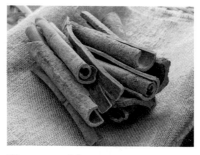

Cinnamon sticks.

Sovereign medicinal herb: cinnamon stick (9 grams). It is Pungent-Sweet and Warm, warming up the meridians and freeing the movement of Yang. It releases the exterior and expels the Coldness.

Minister medicinal herb: white peony root (9 grams). It is Bitter and Sour, and of a slightly Cold nature. It has the function of astringing Yin and strengthening the Blood. Cinnamon sticks expel and white peony root astringes. The combination of the two can expel the pathogenic factor by harmonizing the muscles and skins.

Assistant medicinal herb: ginger (9 grams). It is warm and helps the cinnamon release the exterior and dispel pathogenic factors. It is effective in strengthening the Yang Qi. Alternatively, Jujube (3 to 6 pieces) are effective for this purpose. Dates are Sweet and Warm and help the white peony root nourish the Blood, while white peony root helps to hold the cinnamon in check so that the patient doesn't sweat too much.

Guide medicinal herb: fried licorice root (6 grams). This harmonizes the above herbs.

In the January 2019 issue of *National Geographic*, an article entitled "How Traditional Healing Methods Change Modern Medicine," reported that TCM methods that had long been overlooked by Western medicine were used to generate cutting-edge treatment plans. The article noted that Professor Zheng Yongqi and his team from Yale University had successfully extracted from TCM herbs a drug called PHY906, which could be used for treating cancer. This example points out the important role TCM will play in the future medical practice. PHY906 comes from the scutellaria decoction recorded in the *Treatise on Cold Damage*. The scutellaria decoction is for clearing the bowels, stopping diarrhea and abdominal pain, and soothing anal burning sensations. The formula contains 9 grams of scutellaria as the sovereign herb, 6 grams of white peony as the minister herb, 6 grams of fried licorice root as the assistant herb, and 3 to 5 jujube, depending on the size. This is the source formula for all other treatments for *li* (i.e. diarrhea, *li* referring in ancient times to diarrhea caused by bacteria or a virus). Professor Zheng and his team used this formula to lower the side effects of chemotherapy for liver cancer. In March 2018, the US FDA authorized PHY906 as a valid stand-alone drug for treating liver cancer. The US Cancer Center granted millions of dollars to fund the research on PHY906. This was the first time the Center supported research into treating cancer with TCM herbs.

Professor Zheng praised the theory of sovereign, minister, assistant, and guide herbs, believing that the combination of four herbs is reasonable. If any is removed, the formula will no longer be able to reduce the side effects of chemotherapy. Based on the severeness of the symptoms, the proportion of white peony and licorice root can be 1:1, 3:1, or 6:1.[1]

This application expands the scope of treatment of TCM formulas and opens new paths for the development of TCM. As we have seen, prescription does not merely involve putting several herbs together, but rather forms an integral organic system based on abundant clinical experience. The core of Chinese culture is balance and harmony. Through thousands years of practice and accumulation of experience, doctors have developed and perfected enormous numbers of formulas. They are the treasures of TCM, and the torch should be passed on.

The Variation and Types of Formulas

From this, it is evident that the importance of matching herbs according to a specific formula is meant to enable those herbs to work together in order to better treat the disease while also removing toxins or at least keeping their effects to a minimum. If we use the same herbs in different proportions, even to the point

---

[1] The latest SCI thesis "The Four-Herb Chinese Medicine PHY906 Reduces Chemotherapy-Induced Gastrointestinal Toxicity" in *Science Translational Medicine*, 18 August 2010, Vol 2, Issue 45, pp. 45–59.

of changing which is sovereign and which is minister through the increase or decrease of the ingredients, it will lead to a corresponding change in the function of the formula and the ailments it can treat. Using the cinnamon stick decoction above as a sort of case study, if an increase in the amount of white peony to 18 grams and the amount of sugar to 30 grams will create a new formula, the Minor Center-Fortifying Decoction, which is used to warm the inside of the body. The sovereign then becomes the sugar, which warms the center and nourishes weak Qi, while the cinnamon is relegated to the role of minister, warming the inside and expelling Coldness. The white peony, likewise serving as minister, is good for Yin and nourishes Blood, harmonizing Yin and Yang. The assistant is ginger and dates. Ginger is spicy, and when combined with sweet herbs, it can invigorate Yang. Date is sweet, and when combined with Sour herbs, it can generate Yin. The licorice root complements the Qi and harmonizes the rest of the herbs.

The physical form of an herbal medicine is called the dosage form. Driven by the current clinical needs, many new dosage forms have been developed over the years. There are decoctions, liquors, teas, distillates, pills, powders, pastes, pellets, tablets, lozenges, and capsules to be taken orally and bandages and threads to be used externally. These dosage forms are made by special processes and can be absorbed into the body in the way that most effectively provides healing for a given condition.

With the constraints of space a volume such as this one will inevitably face, I will limit this introduction of matching principles and dosage form to a discussion of decoctions, distillates, pills, and pastes, offering examples of each.

1. Decoction

A decoction is the soup made from boiling herbs. An example is a decoction made from poria, cinnamon twigs, atractylodes macrocephala, and licorice. This decoction is used for treating excessive Phlegm caused by insufficient middle Yang (Yang Qi of the middle energizer of the stomach and spleen). It warms Yang and strengthens the spleen, promoting water movement and dissolving Dampness.

Imbalance (symptoms): chest and ribs filled up with Phlegm, dizziness and palpitations, slippery white tongue coating (Yang weakness with water retention).

Ingredients: 12 grams of poria, as the sovereign herb, which has the function of eliminating Dampness and promoting water, offsetting the offense and reducing the inverse, 9 grams of cinnamon stick as the minister herb, with the function of warming Yang and generating Qi, 9 grams of atractylodes macrocephala koidz, as the assistant herb, which strengthens the spleen and expels Dampness through its bitter warm nature, 6 grams of licorice root as the guide herb, which harmonizes the herbs and complements the Qi.

Procedure: make into decoction. Decoction is primarily used for medicinal herbs, such as roots and bark, though it can have wider applications. When cooking, wash the ingredients thoroughly, chopping into small pieces if necessary, and put into a pot to cook. Add cold fresh water at a ratio of 8–10:1 (water to dry ingredients). After soaking for a half hour, place the pot on the stove and bring to a boil, reducing heat after 2 minutes to the lowest setting. Most herbal decoctions need to be boiled a second time. In the second round, the formula should be allowed to simmer for 10 to 20 minutes. Herbal decoctions should generally boil for 30 minutes, though you should follow any specific directions given in the recipe. Fifteen minutes is sufficient for a small quantity of leaves or flowers, or for a recipe for acute flu or cold. For decoctions with roots or larger items, 30 to 45 minutes is usually required. When finished, strain the decoction and preserve the liquid. If seeds or other materials pass through the strainer, use a fine strainer, again preserving the liquid. Split into multiple portions if necessary and drink warm.

Usage: divide the herbs into 2 portions, drinking one portion in the morning and the other in the afternoon.

Term: 3 days.

2. Distillate

A distillate is the liquid that comes from steaming herbs. An example is the distillate of honeysuckle, which is used for treating heat stroke, rash, and swelling caused when Summer-Heat inflames the lungs and stomach. This distillate clears the Heat and dissolves the toxins.

Imbalance (symptoms): hot and thirsty, sore and swollen throat, fresh red rash, boils, and swelling of the scalp (Heat type)

Ingredients: honeysuckle

Procedure: put 500 grams of honeysuckle in a container and

make 2,000 ml of distillate using the steam distillation method.

Usage: 60 ml 2 to 3 times a day for 1 week

3. Pill

A pill is a ball-shape medicine made from ground herbs mixed with water and honey. The powder is bound together with rice paste. Depending on the adhesive used, the drug can be classified as a water-based pill, honey pill, paste pill, and so forth.

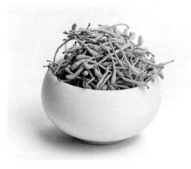

Honeysuckle.

They are easy to take and easy to transport. An example is the giant hawthorn pill, which is a common medicine used for treating indigestion caused by the cumulation of food and distension. It promotes appetite and accelerates the digestion of meat.

Imbalance (symptoms): poor appetite, distension of upper and lower abdomen

Ingredients: Chinese hawthorn berry 100 g, cooked medicated leaven 15 g, cooked malt 15 g

Procedure: make into pills. To thoroughly dry various herbs that are ground into powder, mix evenly and add water or honey to knead into soft dough, then make into small or medium pills.

Usage: 9 g 1 to 2 times a day for 2 days

4. Paste

There are two types of pastes, one for internal and the other for external use. To make a paste for internal use, it is necessary to cook the herbs and make a tonic. After removing the dregs, the tonic is cooked over low heat until it becomes thick. Then rock sugar and honey are added to form a paste.

Pastes for internal use are convenient and their dosage is smaller than tonics. They are often used as complements for treating chronic diseases and are thus taken over a long period. Health maintenance and body nourishment in TCM theory emphasize the importance of nourishing Yin in autumn and winter, complementing in winter and draining in spring. Most prescriptions for nourishing the Yin and complementing Qi take the form of paste. There are overall nourishing pastes that are good for the Qi and Blood, as well as customized pastes for individual patients, which are all very popular.

External paste is also called plaster. To make a plaster, we fry the herbs in vegetable oil such as sesame or rapeseed oil and remove the dregs, then add yellow lead and wax to form paste. It is half solid when cooled down and will melt again when heated. The melted paste is then spread on paper or cloth and applied to the ailing part of the body. If necessary, it can be complemented with other powders. Plaster is normally used for external problems such as rheumatism or injuries.

Example 1: External injury paste consisting of puccoon 120 g, sanguisorba 120 g, gardenia 200 g, rhubarb root 100 g, and other herbs to clear Heat and release toxins. It cools down the Blood, relieves bruises, soothes swelling, and generates muscle growth. It is used to treat traumatic injuries and other skin, muscle and ligament injuries, as well as bone fractures or dislocations. It should be applied externally. Depending on the severity of the injury, the paste can be applied with gauze once a day or once every three days for six to nine days.

Example 2: Sichuan fritillaria and pear syrup for treating weakness in Yin and lung Heat. It nourishes the lungs and eliminates coughs, generating Body Fluids and promoting throat recovery.

Imbalance (symptoms): cough, shortness of breath, dry mouth and throat

Ingredients: watery pear paste 400 g, Sichuan fritillaria 50 g, ophiopogon tuber 100 g, lily bulb 50 g, tussilago 25 g

Procedure: When making the paste, the total weight of the ingredients should be at least 500 to 750 g, with 50 g of each item. To make a paste, follow the same basic procedure as for making a decoction, washing, boiling, straining, then repeating the process. For the first round, the ratio of water to ingredients is 6:1. After the first boil, strain the liquid and keep it separate. Add water to the original ingredients at a 5:1 ratio and boil again. Strain and add the new liquid to the previous amount. Then with a 4:1 ratio, boil, strain, and add this batch to the formerly boiled liquids, discarding all the solid pieces. Use a cloth strainer and strain the combined liquid once more. Place the strained liquid in a cooking pot and reduce further over medium heat. Once the water has mostly boiled off and become sticky, add honey to taste. Allow to cool and store in a glass or ceramic container in the refrigerator. For most pastes, take 1 tablespoon a day, spreading it on toast or adding to hot water for a syrupy drink.

Usage: 15 g twice a day for 2 weeks

Example 3: Sichuan fritillaria and loquat paste is made by combining both fruits and leaves with Sichuan fritillaria, apricot kernel, and other herbs. Mix the paste with 10 ml warm water and drink or eat as a cough drop. Loquat lozenges are also used in TCM for soothing the throat in the early stages of a sore throat or cough.

Other types of commonly used TCM herbs include *xi gua shuang* aerosol spray 西瓜霜喷剂 for treating mouth ulcers, *xi lei san* 锡类散, *ren dan* 人丹, and *shi di shui* 十滴水 for treating heat stroke, Chinese essential balm and cooling ointments for treating headaches and insects stings and keeping warts under control. These are all readily made TCM medicines and are convenient and effective. If you are ever in China, don't forget to bring some home for your friends and family members.

You may refer to Appendix Six for more examples of prescription categorizations.

Chapter Eighteen
Control of the Breath

In Chinese Medicine, control of the breath, is called *tu na*, a special method of inhaling and exhaling. It was generated by vast life experience and healthy activities in the early stages of human civilization in ancient times. The *tu na* method is known as *dantian* breath (*dantian* refers to the upper pubic region) developed in the Qin, Han, and Three Kingdoms periods (221 BC–AD 280). People now call it deep breathing or abdominal breathing. It moves energy from the chest to the abdomen. Usually, we automatically breathe 16 to 18 times per minute. It is a balance between our heart and lungs. One breath is equal to 4 to 5 heartbeats. This follows the natural rhythm of breathing, and when we exercise, swim, feel stressed, in sleep, or feel relaxed, our

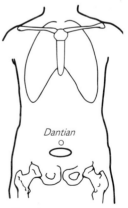

Dantian.

breathing rhythm changes. If we add the mental consciousness and focus (or control) of our breathing to the natural rhythms, we can achieve better health results. Chinese medicine notes that the lung is responsible for producing energy for itself and the whole body. The lungs and the kidney are major organs that cooperate to make breathing complete and efficient. Breathing exercises are a specific part of Chinese Qigong exercises like Tai Chi or Ba Duan Jin.

The Concept and Mechanism

In traditional Chinese culture, Qi is a fundamental concept and is a part of everything that exists. It is everywhere in the universe. Everything you can see, feel, and experience contains Qi. It is created from oxygen that is inhaled during the breathing process, from food essence, and the Original Qi that you are born with.

Almost immediately after birth, a baby will take his or her first breath. Respiration is a natural process that requires no planning or thinking. From childhood through adulthood, our breathing rate starts from being fast, then slows and gradually stabilizes.

Your lungs are the intermediary organ between your internal body and the external environment. When you inhale, your lung Qi should go down and in (descending). When you breathe out, your lung Qi should go up and out (dispersing). In this way, the process of respiration influences all Qi production and movements within the body. The lungs are the organs that govern respiration and dominate Qi. *Basic Questions* says, "The Qi of heaven is in communication with the lungs."

Your kidneys also play a part in respiration. When the lungs take in oxygen, the body needs to cooperate with the kidney to create deeper breathing. When you inhale, kidney energy comes up and attempts to meet the lungs' energy. Once this happens, the kidney energy pulls the Qi down and draws it into itself. If you breathe deeply, the kidney will be more successful in bringing this energy down. The kidney controls the "receiving of Qi." Respiration depends not only on the descending function of the lungs, but also on the kidneys' reception and control. Only when the kidney Qi is strong can the passage of Qi in the lungs be free and the respiration smooth and even. The book *Categorized Patterns with Clear-Cut Treatments* by Lin Peiqin states, "The lungs govern Qi and the kidneys are its root."

Why Do We Need Proper Breath

The lungs play a very important role in this process because the breathing processes enrich the Qi. Without good breathing habits, the quality and quantity of Qi can be affected.

Proper breathing is essential for the lung system and the entire body. Oxygen is used in different physiological functions and is essential to survival. Any disturbance to breathing will eventually affect the whole body.

As we get older, however, we often begin to develop disordered breathing patterns, such as shallow breathing and holding the breath when we are stressed or completing a difficult task. These unhealthy breathing patterns can affect the lung Qi and the total amount of Qi within your system. This is one reason meditation can be an important tool for regulating breathing and affecting one's health. Breathing properly also helps regulate the autonomic nervous system, further promoting the health of the whole body. Deep and diaphragmatic breathing helps you move from a sympathetic nervous system state (fight and flight) to a parasympathetic nervous system state (rest and digest). Shallow breathing and patterns of retaining stress further encourages a hyper-sympathetic nervous system and contribute to the over-production and over-use of hormones such as cortisol and adrenaline. The lungs are the main site for air (oxygen and carbon dioxide) exchange in and out of the body. The alveolar area is generally 60 to 100 square meters. Alveoli are functional units of the lung that are used for air exchange. When one breathes, the alveoli will be subject to some pulling and stimulating effects, lengthening and widening them, making the area larger and the quality of air exchange better. If body posture is not correct or if one is under great stress or does not pay attention to deep breathing, there will be shortness of breath and oxygen will not penetrate into the lower end of the lungs, which will lead to a reduction in the amount of ventilation. Up to 80% or 90% of your lung function during your lifetime depends entirely on how you breathe. There are many ways to breathe, mainly divided into abdominal breathing and chest breathing. If you often sit in the office and don't like sports, breathing will be shorter and shallow, and you will use chest breathing more often. This type of breathing has a small amount of ventilation per breath and insufficient ventilation at normal respiratory rates. It will cause the accumulation of carbon dioxide in the body, leading to hypoxia in the brain and symptoms such as dizziness and fatigue. In order to better take advantage of the potential of your respiratory organs, it is important to consciously slow and deepen your breathing and use abdominal breathing to avoid quick, shallow chest breathing.

Benefits of Combining Chest and Abdominal Breathing

We know that singing and opera are very particular about the use of breath. If the breath and vocal cords cooperate skillfully, not only the volume can be high or low, but also the coherence and vibration of the voice can be guaranteed. The breathing method that most singers admire is called chest and abdominal breathing. It is a holistic activity that coordinates the thorax, diaphragm, and abdominal muscles to achieve maximum control of the breath.

For ordinary people, combining deep breathing with natural chest breathing helps control consciousness, which in turn allows us to further change the rhythm, speed, and depth of our breathing. Deep breathing utilizes the diaphragm and abdomen, increasing the quantity of oxygen and maximizing the quality of movements, which will eventually influence our mental activity and bring more nutrition to our nervous and endocrine systems, encouraging a more relaxed, confident mood and reducing stress. Deep breathing regulates the heartbeat, changes the structure of blood flow, and helps the digestive organs maintain absorption. When we breath deeply, if our posture is correct, the stiffness of the muscle and tendon joints will be corrected, helping to precipitate a sense of inner peace, change secretion of chemical substances, encourage better sleep, and control the early stages of hypertension. Deep breathing can increase the respiratory capacity of our lungs and improve lung functions. (Lung vital capacity refers to the total amount of air that can be inhaled and exhaled after one full effort of breathing.) Most importantly, deep breathing brings an overall state of health, ultimately achieving longevity. In the article "Seeking Vitality Through Breathing," an American scholar points out that practicing deep breathing with control can relieve mental fatigue, regulate the nervous system, and make people more relaxed and comfortable. This is because deep breathing allows one to inhale and exhale 6 to 8 times more Qi than ordinary breathing.[1]

TCM teaches that the lungs control respiration, and with the movement of breath, the oxygen that enters into the body can increase Qi in the organs and meridians, regulate Yin and Yang balance, open and speed up the energy movements along the meridians, and harmonize organ functions for optimal heath. The clinical evidence for breathing exercises shows that it can help reduce pain, stiffness, and symptoms of menopause.

Preparation and Methods of Breath Control
Breathing exercises require an opening of the posture to align the organs and enable the efficient energy exchange between inner body and outside environment. There are two ways of regulating breathing, based on one's normal routine and constitution.

First relax the body from the head to neck, shoulders, chest, abdomen, legs, and toes. The eyes remain open and the tongue touches the upper palate. The legs remain shoulder-width apart.

• Sedentary people should start in a standing position and open the arms away from the body while inhaling through the nose, holding their breath for as long as they can, then exhaling through nose and mouth with the arms returning to the sides. Repeat for several minutes, then follow in a lying posture for 5 to 10 minutes.

• Active people can lie on their back with arms open and palms facing up. Legs should be shoulder-width apart. The toes point outward. As soon as you relax, focus your mind on the respiratory area, inhale from the nose to the belly area, breathing as deep as you can. Hold it as long as you can, then exhale through your mouth as slowly as you can. Repeat 6 times, then return to normal breathing.

After 1 to 2 months of practicing this technique, the heart rate will slowly lower and the breathing rate will gradually slow. After 2 to 3 months of practicing breathing exercise, some people can achieve 3 to 5 breaths per minute, or even 2 to 3 breaths per minute. This is especially true for athletes, such as diving champions, some of whom can be underwater without oxygen mask for 10 minutes. The average people may not be able to achieve such results, but in

---

[1] Hobert, Ingfried, "Healthy Breathing—The Right Breathing" in *Guide to Holistic Healing in the New Millenium*, Munchen: Verlag Peter Erd, 1999, pp. 48–49.

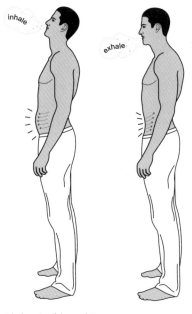

Abdominal breathing.

the conscious training process, breathing 2 or 3 times per minute is still an attainable goal.

One of my clients had a mild case of eczema. The redness on her elbow itched and burned. After practicing these breathing exercises for a week, the redness and itchiness reduced. After a few months, she had completely recovered.

Another client had been diagnosed with hypertension. According to her general practitioner, she needed blood pressure medicine. The TCM diagnosis showed that the root cause was her stressful lifestyle and anxious personality. She started these breathing exercises, and after two months, she was able to keep her blood pressure in the normal range. She combined this breath control with the food therapy and massage.

When practicing, slowly inhale through your nose. During the inhalation process, the thorax is lifted and the abdomen will slowly raise. Continue to inhale until the lungs are completely full of air. At this time, the ribcage will rise and the chest will be enlarged. This process usually takes three seconds. Hold your breath for five seconds before exhaling slowly for two seconds. After exhaling, start a new sequence.

Long-term physical exercise can also improve breathing. For example, swimming can increase people's lung capacity to up to 5,000 to 7,000 ml, well beyond the 3,000 to 4,000 ml of those who do not swim. Long-distance running produces the most obvious increase in maximum oxygen intake. Push-ups can improve the muscle capacity around the chest wall and increase the strength of the respiratory muscles. Lung capacity naturally decreases with aging.

The most critical aspects of respiratory control are:

- Find a comfortable body posture and a quiet place to allow you to focus on breathing.

• Start abdominal breathing. When inhaling, use your nose and expand your belly (place your hand there to monitor it). When exhaling, lead the Qi to the top of the head and exhale with mouth.

• Inhale (deep), hold (5 seconds), and exhale (slow).

This breathing exercise will allow the oxygen to fill the whole area of the alveoli. Moreover, when inhaling, try to make the abdomen bulge, then hold it for 5 to 10 seconds before bringing the oxygen to the abdomen from the upper chambers of the lungs. Exhaling thoroughly will allow the pores to open completely. In this way, all the discarded carbon dioxide can be excreted. This ensures that the alveoli have enough space to inhale oxygen.

This breathing method is called the complete breathing method. It makes muscle groups such as the lungs, ribs, and diaphragm achieve maximum obedience and increases parasympathetic excitability, along with gastrointestinal and rectal movements, which is conducive to digestion and absorption, creating greater fitness and longevity.

When you first start breath control, you can also choose the Qigong stationary standing position (feet shoulder-width apart, knees slightly bent), the sitting position, or the meditation posture. Relax and adjust your breathing. Deep breathing can even be practiced while walking. Each session ranges from 10 to 15 minutes, and perseverance is the only way to maximize effects. At first, you might feel that you cannot find a posture in which your limbs are relaxed, or that your thoughts are clouded or your heart rate is increasing. These are normal phenomena that are often encountered during initial practice. If you persist for a few days, you will improve sleep and focus and feel more relaxed. In your initial practice, you can be guided by a trusted instructor or join a group of students and practice together. It helps to establish good behavioral postures and habits and is conducive to persistence.

Different Focal Points in Breath Control and Meditation

There are many similarities between breath control and meditation. Breath control focuses on breathing, strengthening its length and depth and slowing down its frequency. Meditation maintains a certain posture, meditates quietly, and focuses on emptying the

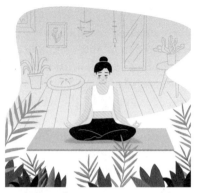

Meditation focuses on emptying the thoughts from the mind.

thoughts from the mind and breathing naturally. Examples of two exercises will demonstrate the difference between breath control and meditation.

Breath exercises to enhance renal function: with the tip of the tongue touching the upper gums and eyes facing upward, slowly inhale while contracting the anus, then hold the position for 10 seconds. Relax while exhaling. Do this 6 to 8 times, increasing the amount of saliva to wash your mouth, slowly swallowing it. This exercise will increase the blood flow to the kidneys and replenish kidney energy and function, enhance the bladder muscles' ability and capacity to control urination, and prevent or treat frequent urination, urinary incontinence, enuresis, and similar conditions.

Six-word meditation exercise: when exhaling, recite the six-word (*xu* for liver system, *he* for heart system, *hu* for spleen system, *si* for lung system, *chui* for kidney system, *xi* for the *sanjiao* system) sounds silently. This is the Taoist method of health care. Using the different force points of the mouth, lips, teeth, throat, and tongue when the pronunciation is used will move the blood of the viscera and meridians. When starting, first vocalize, then gradually transit to silently read a tone without sound. Practice on an empty stomach, and when you exhale, meditate on a tone without sound, then repeat six times. This exercise can help open blockage in the organs.

Chapter Nineteen
Sleep and Meditation

From a physiological perspective, sleep patterns go through different phases in youth, middle age, and old age. Most infants under three have a sleeping pattern in which they sleep early and wake early, and they have a nap after eating lunch. As we enter puberty, we transit to one of two patterns, the early bird or the night owl. Early birds will have an easy time adapting to a typical school or work routine. As we enter middle age or pre-menopause, our sleep pattern changes again. Usually daily allotted sleeping hours will be shortened by an hour or an hour and a half compared to our youth. All these are considered normal changes in life.

TCM View of Sleep Rhythms

TCM categorizes sleep primarily according to heart system functions. Sleep quality and quantity and how one feels when they get up in the morning are areas by which we evaluate whether someone has enough sleep. Since we spend almost a third of our life sleeping, sleep conditions greatly influence our thinking and daily energy.

TCM teaches that our lifestyle should follow the sun. If you happen to be an early bird, this is great, as you're regulating your lifestyle according to the sun. This means that during summer, you wake up earlier than in wintertime. It could be half an hour or one-hour difference. The sun rises later during winter and it sets later, meaning some people may sleep a little later. But during winter, it usually grows dark after 4 or 5 pm, so naturally people should sleep much earlier, before or around 11 pm. You should always consider your individual needs and lifestyle and adjust them according to the sun.

Why Do We Need Enough Sleep

There is a Chinese saying that instructs human beings to keep their vitality and follow the pattern of *ri chu er zuo, ri luo er xi* 日出而作，日落而息 , which means starting one's work at sunrise and resting at sunset. Sleep plays an important role in our mental and physical health and should be of concern to people of all ages. However, many people have various sleeping problems. Many young people like to stay up late, thinking that sleep has little to do with them. In the long run, staying up late and irregular sleep slowly nibble into their energy.

We say that exercise and learning are two ways to secure focus and strength. Energy is the expression of mental and physical health, while sleep is one of its foundations and premises. Sleep can eliminate fatigue, restore physical strength, protect the brain, promote adolescent growth and development, and improve our immunity and appearance. Sleep is one of the most important means of maintaining one's body and youthful appearance.

Modern Research Findings Regarding Sleep

Modern research findings indicate that sleep is regulated by two body systems, sleep/wake homeostasis and the circadian biological clock. The internal circadian biological clocks regulates the timing of sleepiness and wakefulness throughout the day. The circadian rhythm dips and rises at different points during the day, so adults' strongest sleep drive generally occurs between 2:00 to 4:00 am and in the afternoon between 1:00 to 3:00 pm, although there is some variation depending on whether you are a "morning person" or "evening person." The sleepiness we experience during these circadian dips will be less intense if we have sufficient sleep and more intense when we are sleep deprived. The circadian rhythm also causes us to feel more alert at certain points of the day, even if we have been awake for hours and our sleep/wake restorative process would otherwise make us feel sleepier.

The glymphatic system (or glymphatic clearance pathway, or paravascular system) is a functional waste clearance pathway for the vertebrate central nervous system (CNS). Maiken Nedergaard, a Danish neuroscientist renowned for discovering the glymphatic system (2012, *Journal of Translational Medicine*), is a jointly appointed professor in the Departments of Neuroscience and Neurology at the University of Rochester Medical Center. After discovering the glymphatic system, researchers have conducted a series of experiments on mice to better understand how the system works and when it is most active. This team is particularly concerned about the connections between sleep and Alzheimer's disease. The study found that the glymphatic system of the brain is busiest when the animal is sleeping. They found that when the mice slept, the gap increased by 60%. The increase in the size of the gap promotes the exchange of cerebrospinal and interstitial fluids and accelerates the clearance of amyloid. They concluded that the recovery function of sleep might be the result of enhanced clearance of potentially neurotoxic waste accumulated when awake (central nervous system).

In addition to its immune function, the lymphatic system is also responsible for removing metabolic waste from the body. However, there is no lymphoid tissue in the brain parenchyma, so the question of how the brain removes metabolic waste has plagued scientists. A 2012 article in the *Journal of Science in Translational Medicine* first proposed the concept of the glymphatic system stating that the subarachnoid cerebrospinal fluid (CSF) moves along the arterial perivascular space (PVS, same as VRS) in the same direction as the blood flow, then passes through the water channel-4 (AQP4) on the arterial vessel and enters the brain parenchyma, where the cerebrospinal fluid (CSF) exchanges metabolites with the interstitial fluid (ISF) in the brain and the CSF with the metabolite enters the vein through the AQP4 on the venous PVS. Finally, the metabolic waste flows along the venous PVS in the same direction as the blood flow and is excreted. Further studies have shown that sleep is the most active state of the glymphatic system. Currently, a popular hypothesis is that the accumulation of toxins in the brain or the damaged glymphatic system is the cause and progression of most neurodegenerative diseases. It is thus important to go to bed at the appropriate time to ensure quality sleep.

Improving Sleep Quality with TCM

What does good quality sleep mean? Did you sleep like a baby? Like the life cycle, babies sleep soundest, then as they age and mature, they may experience sleep difficulties. Once we become old, we go back to sleeping long and soundly, much like babies. Are you able to do things efficiently? Are you able to get up easily with motivation within 20 minutes of waking? If you find it hard to get up in the morning, your mental and physical body will not work efficiently during the day.

How deep is your sleep? Do you wake up in the middle of the night to use the bathroom? Do you feel energized when you wake up in the morning? Ideally, we do not want to rely on smart watches or electronic devices to tell us how deeply we slept. We should be able to feel this in our own bodies.

There are generally three conditions we need to address to improve sleep quality:

Difficulty falling asleep.

Difficulty sleeping through the night. Most people have 4 to

5 hours of continuous sleep during one phase. Ideally, we want two phases a night, but when we get older we may only get 1.5 phases. How many times do you wake up in the night? Do you wake up to drink water or use the restroom? Some people may even wake up for no reason.

Feeling tired when you wake up. If you wake up two or more times during the night before you are 65 to 70 years old, this is too much. If it happens after the age of 70, it is considered normal.

Here are several ways to address these sleep problems and identify which condition you may experience.

1. According to Different Patterns

Hot condition: if you feel it difficult to fall asleep, it could be that your body is too Hot, or too Yang, and you need to remove some Heat from your body. It could be that you have a busy mind and are thinking too much before you sleep. For this condition, sometimes eating a bit of food before bed to transfer blood from the head to the stomach will make it easier to sleep. This is why traditionally people would drink milk to help them sleep, or millet porridge or lily bulb soup. If eating these foods does not help, then you can try soaking your feet in hot water, as there are more meridians in the feet and this transfers the blood from the head to the feet. These two methods may help you fall asleep more easily. Some people may need melatonin to help with them rest or to recover from jetlag. It provides them with a chemical that regulates sleep.

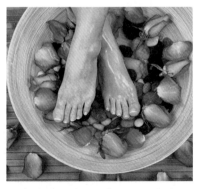

Soaking your feet in hot water before bed can improve sleep quality.

Urinary and digestive issues: if you wake up many times during the night to urinate, it could be that the kidneys have problems. Herbs such as Reishi mushroom and Schisandra berry can be used to help you sleep. People with this issue can also change the way they drink water. For example, if they drink 1.5 liters a day, they should try to finish 70% before dinner, or by 5 pm. At night, they should only have 30% of their daily water consumption. It is best to take no more than 50 ml of water two hours before sleeping. If you drink a large bowl of soup at dinner time, you should not drink much more water unless you feel dehydrated, and even then, only drink 50 to 150 ml at most. Some people feel dry mouth or thirsty easily, but older people with heart issues, hypertension, or thick blood should drink just a mouthful of water each time they wake at night. For younger people, if it is disturbing your sleep, perhaps you should regulate your digestive issues. You can also drink specific teas at night. One well-known tea is made from a gluey millet mixed with pinellia rhizome and cooked as a decoction to prevent and treat insomnia. It also helps harmonize digestion and helps you fall asleep. Another lifestyle change is to avoid eating dinner too late. How many hours each person needs to digest is slightly different. If you sleep at 11 pm, you should finish your dinner before 8 pm. If you have digestive issues, such as stomach discomfort, this can cause you to have trouble sleeping as well. TCM teaches that if the stomach is not in harmony, it will be restless.

Lack of nourishment: another issue is that some people wake up too early and cannot fall asleep again. They end up feeling lethargic during the day. Even with five hours of sleep, they cannot completely address their mental exhaustion. TCM teaches that this is due to liver Heat or Heat in the chest. It could also be due to insufficient fluids, which leaves the body undernourished. Evening sleep time is when Yin energy is predominant, and the daytime is when Yang energy is predominant. If Yang energy enters your body but your Yin energy is able to handle it, you can continue sleeping. If Yang energy is too intense, it will prevent you from sleeping early. It is all about this balance. Too much Yang or too little Yin can cause sleep issues. Less Yin or less nourishment is related to your quantity and quality of Blood, how much water or Body Fluid you have and how strong your organ system is. So, for people who wake up too early, toning Body Fluid and boosting the quantity of the Blood is important. In China, people eat whole oats, walnuts, or boiled peanuts with sea salt to help with sleep. Peanuts are full of oil and are known to tone and help with sleep issues, especially for those who wake too early.

In addition, people can meditate to help them sleep better,

focusing on breathing and being in a state of calmness or quiet, which can nourish Yin energy. Soft, gentle energy is needed for the body to develop more Yin qualities.

2. According to Diagnosis and Lifestyle

There are several types of people who experience sleep difficulties, and they can be roughly divided into three categories.

Insomnia: for patients with insomnia, bedtime preparation is especially important. For those people who have difficulty falling asleep, we recommend "three tips" to improve the quality of sleep.

First, eat less indigestible foods, and avoid having dinner too late. Otherwise, the stomach will feel full and you will not easily fall asleep.

Second, follow appropriate daily sleep patterns in order to form a fixed biological clock.

Third, drink a small quantity (50 to 75 ml) of relaxing flower tea, with 5 g of feverfew or chrysanthemum.

People with irregular lifestyle: people with an irregular life must give themselves a reason to sleep, such as sleep is good for the skin, sound sleep is like giving the skin a free beauty treatment, or often reminding themselves that the current overdraft of their bodies indicates future illnesses that must be paid.

Anxious personality: for patients who suffer from insomnia due to anxiety, the most common experience is that there are many things on their minds that make them constantly worried and anxious. These people may not be able to calm their minds (thinking a lot), they cannot be quiet (heartbeat is fast and heavy), and the body can't calm down (tossing and turning). You can try the "IBM method" to address these issues.

I is for information. The most troubled patients have anxiety and insomnia due to too much information and too many thoughts in the brain. In this case, you can integrate the excess information and write it down. For example, when you fall asleep at night, if you are worried about setting up a venue, vehicle arrangements, or dining arrangements for the following day, you can classify these three things into three keywords, venue, vehicle, and dining, to greatly reduce the amount of information in your mind.

B is for bedtime tea. Brew 5 g of feverfew or 2 g chamomile into a tea. Some may prefer to drink half a glass of red wine.

M is for meditation. Integrate things into several keywords, and if you can't stop thinking about them, lie flat and concentrate on the number of breaths you take. Anxiety, the inability to fall asleep, a rapid, heavy heartbeat, and irritability can be addressed through deep breathing. Take a deep breath, slowly exhale 2 to 3 times in slow succession. Your feelings of chest tightness, rapid heartbeat, and other symptoms will gradually subside into drowsiness.

If you are still worried about sleep, you can try these methods and perhaps you will be surprised with the outcome.

Paying attention to sleep means paying attention to health. If you sleep soundly, you will have good health. It is my hope that young people will pay attention to their sleep patterns, older people will enjoy sleep, and people with insomnia will improve their sleep.

Sit in Meditation

Sitting in meditation is a method of maintaining health and fitness. Sit cross-legged, adjust your breath, put your hands in a certain position, and clear your mind.

Meditation is also called "sitting cross-legged" or "sitting quietly," and is a basic method of cultivation and practice in Taoism. It is also a compulsory course in Buddhism. In Chinese martial arts, meditation is also a way of cultivating internal strength of energy, mind, and perseverance.

Meditation can not only prolong life, but also increase wisdom. Meditation is a static state, according to the Chinese saying, *jiu jing ze ding, jiu dong ze pi* 久静则定，久动则疲 , which means "when you are static, you can make your body and mind stable; frequent and excessive activity can be physically and mentally exhausting." It denotes that static state and movement are similar to Yin and Yang, the sun and the moon, or day and night. It is best to keep a relative balance to transit smoothly and moderately between them in the operative order of life. At the end of a session of quiet meditation, it is important to move your

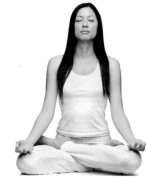

Sitting cross-legged.

muscles and tendons, doing some stretching and self-massage to ensure a dynamic combination.

Ding Fubao (1874–1952) wrote a book at his 70th birthday about methods of obtaining longevity. In the book, he emphasizes the importance of caring for the heart (including the mind) and sitting quietly. Ding was a weak, ill child, and he was very thin with little muscle mass. He was also very short and small. In addition, he suffered from a severe lung disease. Ding knew that this sort of constitution was unlikely to bring him health and longevity. He put all his effort into studying methods for the care and improvement of his physical condition, then practiced them. After he turned 30, his body gradually grew stronger, his brain developed, and learning and study became easy for him. The most important aspect of his health protection regimen was Qigong. Ding's other book *The Gist of Sitting in Meditation* stated that if one can continually practice meditation, it can improve focus, increase willpower, help blood circulation, prevent external factors, and improve body functions, including the heart, nervous system, lungs, stomach, colon, liver, and kidneys. If visceral function can be well maintained, it will not be affected by external ailments and diseases, and then we can live to an old age, perhaps nearly a hundred years.

Ding's method of sitting still involved sitting three times a day, in the morning, at noon, and before going to bed. At first, each session is limited to 30 minutes. You can limit the time depending on your physical condition. After two months, you can gradually increase it until you reach one hour. While sitting, the eyes should be partially closed, the head slightly lowered, and the mouth gently closed. Breathe through the nostrils, quiet, light, and long, without any loud breathing sounds. The legs should be crossed naturally with one on the top of the other. You do not have to sit cross-legged, but can instead sit in a chair and keep your hips, knees, and ankles at 90-degree angles. When you sit still, you should be relaxed from head to toe. Empty the mind, and do not think of anything else. Concentrate on only one place, which is what we call the umbilical *dantian* area. The 3 keys are a comfortable and relaxed position, deep and well-regulated breathing, and a quiet state of mind.

I have also interviewed some practitioners who practice meditation. They say that after real entry into a quiet state, they can

enter into a subconscious state. In this subconscious state, positive
pure energy can be used to resolve stress, lower blood pressure,
and eliminate negative energy, which will enable one to reorganize
their relationship with the environment. It is similar to self-induced
hypnosis. (Hypnosis is a therapy to help human conditions, involving
focused attention, reduced peripheral awareness, and an enhanced
capacity to respond to suggestion. There are cases in which those
who practice self-hypnosis have given up such things as smoking or
have learned to control anxiety.)

Broadly speaking, for sitting in meditation, known as *jing zuo* in
Chinese, one must first know what *jing* (quiet) is and why we should
seek it. It is not just being silent, closing your eyes, and plugging
your ears, but also making yourself concentrate and giving your
spirit input, enabling you to reach the realm of selflessness.

We should aim to reach this *jing* level because the realm of
ecstasy can give us tremendous energy and make us physically and
mentally united. It also connects humans to the power of nature.
This power is very strong, but it will not deplete our body's energy.
On the contrary, it helps us discover and develop our inherent,
continuous health recovery potential.

It is important to find the amnesiac state that suits you.
Anything that makes you focus your concentration should be part of
your meditation. It may be sitting in meditation, painting or playing
the piano, or it may also be a sport such as tennis or table tennis, or
the like.

Chapter Twenty

Tai Chi

Tai Chi, an aerobic martial arts exercise, is combined with specific
breathing exercises to strengthen the diaphragm, improve posture,
and make better use of the body's Qi. Practitioners of different
disciplines often interpret the importance of breathing regulation
and its perceived influence on the mood in a variety of ways.[1]

---

[1] Hobert, Ingfried, "Healthy Breathing—The Right Breathing" in *Guide to Holistic Healing in the New Millenium*, Munchen: Verlag Peter Erd, 1999, pp. 48–49.

Introduction to Tai Chi

Tai Chi, or *taijiquan*, is an ancient technique that involves learning or practicing martial arts. It is one of China's traditional national martial arts. It has a long history, with origins dating back to as early as the Song dynasty. Modern Tai Chi was created more than 300 years ago, in the late Ming and early Qing dynasty. Tai Chi was created and developed from many forms of martial arts. During the Wanli period (1573–1620) of the Ming dynasty, martial artist Wang Zongyue wrote a book entitled *Tai Chi Martial Art Theory*, in which he used the term *taijiquan*. Tai Chi is the perfect combination of martial arts, TCM, and Qigong.

Preserving health through sports and exercise has a long history in China. As early as the Three Kingdoms period (220–280), the ancient Chinese people had already developed exercises to keep healthy, and they could explain why the movements were healthy. Distinguished TCM physician Hua Tuo (?–208) created an exercise technique called the Five Animal Style. The five movements were called tiger, deer, bear, monkey, and bird. The techniques were named after these animals because the movements used looked like those of the animals. Hua Tuo observed animals and followed their movements. He believed that these actions were good for humans, especially their joints, spine, and breathing. He claimed that by absorbing the essence of ancient physical and breathing exercises, he mimicked the movements and postures of animals, then created the Five Animal Style.

Today, Tai Chi combines many different movements and has many different variations and styles. It joins form with movement and breathing exercises. Each movement has a specific breathing technique. Tai Chi not only strengthens muscles and joints, but also strengthens the internal organs, especially the lungs and the heart. It strengthens and calms the mind as well, producing a sense of peace in body and mind. Tai Chi brings harmony from the outside world into the body, promoting harmony of the soul. It balances Yin and Yang, as there is a balance of motion and stillness within the practice, and it attunes the body inside and out. The movement of the joints and spine and increased breathing capacity not only contribute to better health, but can also prevent and cure some illnesses and promote agelessness.

Benefits of Tai Chi

In the last 100 years, Tai Chi has spread widely throughout China. People have extensively reviewed and studied all its styles and practices. There is a national Tai Chi practice because it has been proven to improve the physical constitution. As one practices Tai Chi, he or she will become sick less often. After practicing Tai Chi for some time, they notice a reduction in symptoms of prior illnesses, pain, and joint stiffness. It also promotes longevity and is considered to be anti-aging and to engender happiness. As a result, after 1949, Tai Chi was taught as a part of physical education classes in schools in China. When I was a young girl in middle and high school, Tai Chi was taught in my P.E. classes.

Before 1949, there were only a few Traditional Chinese Medicine colleges. After that time, however, every province had a TCM college or university. All these colleges taught Tai Chi as part of the physical education curriculum. The schools also taught Tai Chi to the community on weekends or as continuing education courses. Because Tai Chi was taught to the general public at the TCM schools, it became popular. Tai Chi is sometimes referred to as TCM's medicinal physical education.

Tai Chi has been studied by medical researchers, who found that it influences the nervous system, cardiovascular system, respiratory system, digestive system, and the metabolism. It has a positive influence on all bodily systems. While practicing Tai Chi, the mind focuses on the changes and movements of the limbs, while the eyes follow the movement of the hands and fingers. The spine or trunk moves first, and the feet follow. All the movements form a circle. The circular movements are fluid, flexible, and smooth. The left and right side of the body are always balanced. If a movement is practiced using the left side of the body, the same movement is practiced with the right side of the body. In Tai Chi, movements go from one side of the body to the other, from left to right or right to left, smoothly changing and balancing the two sides of the body. These movements are good for brain response and function, and they change the practitioner's reactions to the environment. The movements utilize the left and right sides of the brain, and the two sides of the brain interact positively and peacefully.

Tai Chi is sometimes referred to as shadow boxing in English.

The term boxing can be misleading, as Tai Chi is very different from the fighting sport of boxing with fists. It is slow, uses soft movements, and is always accompanied with music. The rhythm of the music is needed in order to create a rhythm for the muscles and joints to stretch and contract, while also building up muscular strength. It is particularly good for weak or atrophied muscles. Tai Chi is good for the sympathetic nervous system too, as it improves balance and coordination. Coordination improves because links between the meridians or nerves and the organs are built up. Qi moves from organs to meridians, then back to the organs.

Tai Chi is recommended for middle aged people and seniors, and for people who suffer from chronic illnesses because it increases the body's capacity to rehabilitate, stabilize illness, and enhance quality of life. It is even safe for seniors. Tai Chi is a good source of exercise for the elderly. It is an exercise that is energy-building, not energy-taking, and is viewed as an energy tonic.

It is typically practiced in the sunlight, often in a nice garden or a place with a pleasurable atmosphere, and soothing music is played. It is usually practiced with friends or with a community. In China, many people practice Tai Chi in parks or nice green spaces near their homes. Some people find a Tai Chi teacher or master to practice with and learn from. Once they have learned the basics, they can continue to practice on their own or with videos. If one cannot go to a park to practice, he or she can often practice in their community clubhouse or other convenient locations. People who practice Tai Chi discover their own reasons for practicing and enjoying its unique benefits, and with regular practice, most people experience the many benefits discussed above.

Application of Tai Chi
These six movements are commonly introduced to beginners of Tai Chi.

1. **Cloud Hands** (左右云手 *zuo you yun shou*)

Preparation: stand with feet shoulder-width apart, parallel and facing forward. Relax and bend both knees enough to relax, drop and tuck in the tailbone slightly. The arms are by the sides in a relaxed manner. The shoulders are relaxed. Gaze directly forward, not up or down. The head should be in the most relaxed position. The tongue should touch the roof of the mouth behind the upper front teeth.

Left Cloud Hand: from the preparation position, weight moves onto the right leg. The left hand rises up from the hips across the front of the abdomen to the right, in front of the shoulder, palm facing the body. Then the weight transfers onto left leg and the left arm extends out from body and to the left until it is extended in front of the left shoulder, with the eyes always following the left hand. The inside of the palm opens to the left. As the left hand begins to open to the left and is still close to the trunk, the right hand moves up from the hips in front of the body. The movement finishes with right hand in front of the body near the left shoulder and left hand extended in front of the left shoulder. The eyes follow the left hand because the left side produces the lead motion. Do not look at the right hand, but keep the right elbow slightly bent. This motion is round, resembling a cloud. The movements should be slow and fluid.

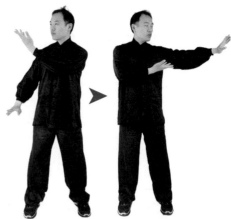

Left Cloud Hand.

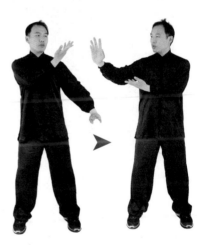

Right Cloud Hand.

To complete the movement and balance the body's Yin and Yang, after Left Cloud Hand we will have Right Cloud Hand, the sequence is from left to right.

Right Cloud Hand: the movements are the same as Left Cloud Hand, but in the opposite direction. The eyes follow the right hand.

Cloud Hands can be practiced many times. Move back and forth from left to right 10 to 20 times, with the eyes always following the leading hand.

2. Parting the Wild Horse's Mane (左右分鬃 *zuo you fen zong*)
Preparation: the same with Cloud Hands.

Left Parting the Mane: from the preparation position, the body weight shifts onto the right leg. The arms move in front of the body, as if holding a large beach ball. The right hand moves up in front of the body to chest level, not too high and with the palm facing down. The right hand holds the top of an imaginary ball. At the same time, the left hand moves up to the bottom of the belly, palm facing up, holding the bottom of the ball. There should be a roundness to the movements.

As the weight moves onto left leg, the arms enlarge the ball.

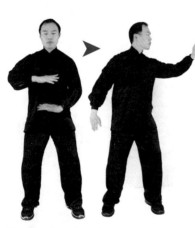

Left Parting the Mane.

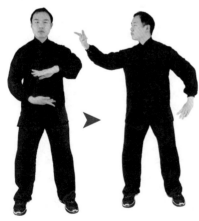

Right Parting the Mane.

To move onto the left leg, turn the body to the left at about a 45-degree angle, while bending and stepping the left leg to the left and transferring the weight onto the left, like shooting an arrow. When the weight is on the left leg, the arms follow. The left arm moves up from the belly button to the right, in front of the body with the palm facing up. Once the left hand is in front of the right shoulder, the left arm moves out, away from the body and to the left, in a flowing, circular motion, palm facing up. At the same time, the right arm moves from the middle of the chest to the right hip in a circular motion, palm facing down. This is the mane parting action. The eyes follow the left hand, as it is the leading arm in this movement.

When the weight is on the left leg and the arms are extended, move back to center, following the same plan as the extension and holding another imaginary ball in the center, with the weight on the right leg and arms extended.

With every movement to left or right, first hold the ball in center. If moving to the left, left palm facing up, holding the bottom of the ball, or if moving to the right, right palm facing up, holding the bottom of the ball. Once you have the ball, move to the left or right.

Right Parting the Mane: to complete the movement and balance the body's Yin and Yang, the sequence is performed to the right with the same movements. First the weight shifts onto the left leg, left arm back, left palm facing down in the upper level and right palm facing up, holding the bottom of the ball. The right arm moves up and to the right, eyes following the right hand. The left arm moves to the left hip, palm facing down.

Parting the Mane can be practiced many times. Move back and forth from left to right 10 to 20 times, with the eyes always following the lead arm.

3. **Brush Knee** (左右搂膝 *zuo you lou xi*)

Preparation: the same with Cloud Hands.

Left Brush Knee: stand with feet shoulder-width apart, parallel and facing forward. The left hand moves up to the right side of the chest, palm facing down, towards the body. At the same time, the right hand moves up the right side of the body to ear level and the right arm bends at the elbow, palm facing upward. The body weight moves onto the right leg. Bend the right knee to take the weight. The left hand moves from the chest and swoops down to brush the left knee, then swoops up to the left hip, palm facing the floor. At the same time, the right hand moves from the ear and extends

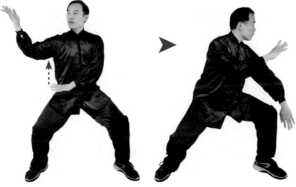

Left Brush Knee.

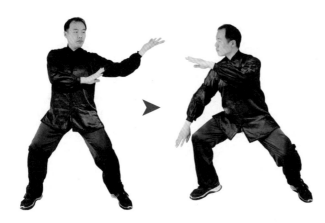

Right Brush
Knee.

out from the body at the same level as the nose, to a comfortable
45-degree angle. The eyes follow the right hand, the leading arm
in movement, not the left hand. In this movement, the left knee is
brushed, but most of the body weight is on the right leg.

Right Brush Knee: move back to the starting position, this
time with right hand in front of the left chest and the left hand
up and to the left ear. To complete the movement and balance
the body's Yin and Yang, the sequence is performed to the right,
with body weight moving onto the left leg, the right hand swoops
down to brush the right knee. The eyes follow the left hand. The
movement is the same as the left side, but in the opposite direction.

Brush Knee can be practiced many times. Move back and forth
from left to right 10 to 20 times, with the eyes always following the
leading hand.

First practice these exercises to gain a feel for Tai chi and its
smooth, fluid movements. To further your practice, find a Tai Chi
master or teacher near you or watch instructional videos online. Tai
Chi's 24 Forms is a good starting place for beginners, but even these
six basic movements, practiced 20 minutes a day, can yield benefits.

Chapter Twenty-One
Ba Duan Jin

Ba Duan Jin (literally 8 pieces of brocade) is a set of eight Qigong
exercises with medical benefits. There are two interesting and

meaningful reasons why the word *jin* 锦 was chosen to describe these exercises. First, *jin* means brocade, a colorful, elaborate woven fabric often displayed as wall hangings in China. *Jin* also means bright and beautiful. A silken brocade takes a very long time to make. It is beautiful, delicate, soft, and precious. *Jin* was used to describe the 8 sections because it was thought that the exercises embody these characteristics and impart them on the practitioner. The other reason *jin* was chosen is that for each section, the physical movements and the breathing exercises are woven continuously like silk threads, eventually creating a complete picture.

Introduction to Ba Duan Jin

Ba Duan Jin began in the Northern Song dynasty, more than 800 years ago. Since it is called 8 segments or 8 pieces, meaning there are 8 different exercise sequences, each piece is independent of the others, but all 8 segments together are complete and well organized for the entire body system. Each piece targets one area of the body.

Ba Duan Jin is simple health care Qigong. The practice is easy to learn. It can be practiced anywhere and does not require any equipment. One can practice 2 or 3 segments, or all 8, repeating each segment 6 times each time. Because each movement targets a specific area of the body, one can choose to practice the exercise that targets their weaker organ systems. It is suitable for both males and females, young and old, and those with large or slim builds. It can help thin people build up body strength and heavier people reduce weight. After practicing regularly for some time, one will notice significant results in the organ systems. Ba Duan Jin can treat and prevent some illnesses.

The content of Ba Duan Jin has changed slightly since ancient times. For example, the national principle of Ba Duan Jin and that practiced in the community is slightly different. Ba Duan Jin has developed into two main styles. The Northern Style is a seated style. However, seated style in this case refers to the standing position in which the knees are deeply bent, as if sitting on a horse. The Northern Style is a stronger, quicker, and more powerful version of Ba Duan Jin. It is usually practiced by young and middle-aged people and is considered to be more of a martial art and is practiced competitively. The Southern Style is softer and gentler and is practiced in a standing position. It is suitable for the elderly or weaker individuals. Both styles are derived from the same origins.

An important discovery for Qigong was made in the Mawangdui Ancient Tomb in Changsha, Hunan Province of China. In ancient times, people were buried with some of their important possessions, such as art pieces and even medicine. The 44 *daoyin* (health-care Qigong) movements depicted on a silk painting were found in the Mawangdui Tomb. Several movements were somewhat similar to the Five Animal's Style and Ba Duan Jin movements. It is not known exactly by whom or when the paintings were created. Based on the pictures, historians believe that health care workers or rehabilitation specialists, like modern day physiotherapists, worked together with marital artists to create the Ba Duan Jin Qigong exercises.

Three Levels of Ba Duan Jin

Ba Duan Jin existed before the Song dynasty but was named in the Song dynasty. Pictures and principles of the movements developed and spread quickly during the Ming and Qing dynasties. Before the Qing dynasty, the focus was on the movement of the body, with less focus on breathing and moving Qi. After the Qing dynasty, people learned more about anatomy and consciousness, learning that mental wellness, consciousness, and the body were all linked. They studied body structure and meridians and practiced deep breathing, then added body movements to the breathing. They found that by breathing and moving the body, one could achieve relaxation that would move from consciousness to the Qi and to the body, creating harmony among consciousness, breath, and body. Eventually some people achieved relaxation of the highest spiritual mind or soul, or *ling* 灵 in Chinese. Few people can attain relaxation of the highest spiritual level. The middle or second level is the mind or consciousness (*jing shen* 精神). It is believed that if one has good consciousness, they will also have good health. It is much easier to achieve relaxation of this level, and it is thus possible for more people. The lowest and third level is emotion (*qing xu* 情绪). One can be moody or emotional but still have good consciousness. By practicing Ba Duan Jin, the body relaxes, emotions are calmed, and one can achieve relaxation of the second level or relaxation of the mind and consciousness. Many people practice Ba Duan Jin because it helps them relax. One can concentrate on relaxing the mind, then begin the movements, or one can start with the bodywork and find that they become more relaxed and begin to concentrate. With the body movements and adjustment of the breathing, relaxation can come to the mind or consciousness. Ba Duan Jin is flexible. One can adjust it to suit their needs. For example, one can choose to do large movements or small movements, to stand or bend the knees deeply and sit low, or to repeat the exercises six or eight times. It all depends on one's personal needs and condition.

Application of Ba Duan Jin

The Yellow Emperor's Internal Canon of Medicine holds that the most fundamental factor in the internal causes of human aging is the degeneration of vitality in the kidneys. If we can maintain the function and adjust the balance of Yin and Yang in the kidneys, it will be effective in delaying aging and prolonging life. The digestive system, represented by the spleen and stomach, belongs to the earth element. Earth is the mother of all things. In TCM, the spleen and stomach are called the root of the acquired constitution, the source of Qi and Blood. The *sanjiao* connects and communicates with the whole visceral and is a passage for circulating the Original Qi and Body Fluids (including lymph liquid). Therefore, it is advisable to start with the following three pieces in your practice.

1. **Piece 3: Spleen**

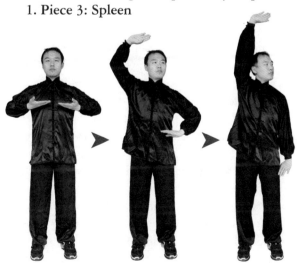

Piece 3: spleen.

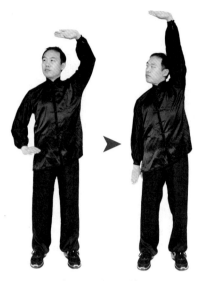

Piece 3: spleen (continued).

Raise the hands to condition the stomach and spleen, separating heaven and earth. To regulate the spleen and stomach, one must balance the upper and lower extensions of the arms.

Preparation: stand with feet shoulder-width apart, parallel and facing forward. Bend both knees enough to relax, and drop and tuck in the tailbone slightly. The arms should be at the sides of the body in a relaxed manner. The shoulders are relaxed. Gaze directly forward, not up or down. The head should be in the most relaxed position. The tongue should touch the roof of the mouth behind the upper front teeth.

To begin, move both arms up slightly in front of the body to about chest level, palms softly cupped and facing up. From the center of the body, the right hand slowly moves upward in front of the body, as if the palm is collecting energy. Once the hand is in front of the head, the palm slowly turns to face the sky as the arm extends fully above the shoulder. The right arm should be fully extended, palm facing the sky and fingers pointing in towards the head. At the same time the left arm extends down to the right hip. Fully extend the left arm, palm facing down, fingers facing forward, and unbend both knees. Both arms begin by extending at the same time and moving at the same smooth pace. Once both arms are fully extended, hold the pose for a few seconds. Both arms gently move back to the center of the body to the starting position. To complete the movement and balance the body's Yin and Yang, the sequence is performed with the left hand extending up and the right extending down. Repeat 6 times. After a few days, you will feel the Qi inside your palm.

This exercise follows the natural movements of the stomach and spleen. TCM believes stomach Qi moves down and spleen Qi moves up. This exercise helps send pure energy up from the spleen to support and nourish the head and sensory organs. Repeating the up

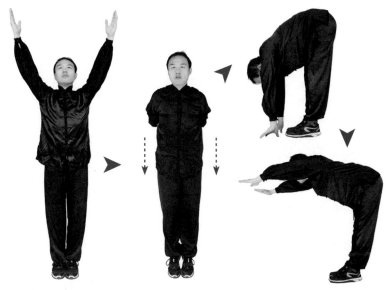

Piece 6: kidney.

and down movements regulates and harmonizes the function of the digestive system.

2. Piece 6: Kidney

Both hands touch the lower back and lower limbs in order to strengthen the kidneys.

Preparation: same as piece 3.

At the same time, both arms extend out and move upward in front of the body, palms facing down, until the arms are fully extended above the head and shoulders with palms facing forward.

Once the arms are fully extended above the head, the arms move down, the elbows bend, and the hands and fingers point inward towards each other. The hands move down in front of the face to chest level. Then the hands turn, palms face up, and move into the body, under the armpits. The hands then move along the sides of the body to the back, palms touching the body. The hands touch the back of the body with the fingers pointing down. The hands press the body from the back of the ribs all the way down the back of the body and the back of the legs to the feet. The hands then move around the sides of the feet and over the top of the feet to touch the toes. At same time, bend from the waist, keeping the knees straight

235

if possible. The movement finishes at the toes. To finish the exercise, the body moves back to the preparation position. Repeat 6 times.

This exercise regulates the kidneys. In TCM, the back is considered the home of the kidneys. The meridians of the urinary bladder and the kidneys finish and start from the feet. In this exercise, one moves the hands along the Bladder Meridian points. The back and spine are considered the axis of the body. The back is linked with the kidney system. This section strengthens the back and kidney function. It is especially helpful for constipation and back pain, as it strengthens the lower back and lower abdominal muscles. If one has hypertension or a cardiovascular illness, gently lower the head, taking care not to lower it too much.

3. Piece 8: Entire Body/Back & Spine

Shake the back seven times to relieve 100 illnesses, moving the heels up and down and bouncing on the toes.

Preparation: same as piece 3.

Cup fingers together softly, palms facing the hips, fingers facing down, and arms hanging loosely beside the body. You can also place your hands on both sides of your lower back to support your body. The heels lift up, weight moving up and into the toes. The hands drift slightly upward, the elbows bend slightly, and the upper back moves up a little. Quickly drop all of the body weight onto the heels as the shoulders drop. Repeat 6 times.

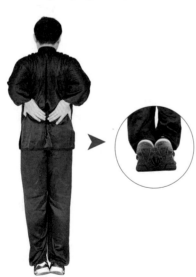

Energy moves from the heels through the spine to the head, creating a vibration. The vibration moves through the whole body, massaging the central and sympathetic nervous systems and the Governing Vessel, relaxing body and mind. This is good for blood circulation, removes or aids recovery from fatigue, and regulates the organ systems. Long term regular practice of this exercise can

Piece 8: entire body.

strengthen the constitution and remove some illnesses. In the eighth segment, the whole body is targeted, because the spine and back are important for the entire body, both inside and outside.

Since this set of exercises is simple, easy to follow and practice, it has long been popular and produced satisfactory results. Many TCM professors also practice it throughout their lives for general health care. You can start by repeating a few movements which can improve your weak or unbalanced organs.

Chapter Twenty-Two
Healthy Lifestyle: Regulation of Daily and Seasonal Rhythms, Life Stages and Space

Lifestyle refers to one's patterns in daily life, including the basic necessities such as how and what to eat, how to dress, how to balance work, exercise, and leisure time, and other such factors. A healthy lifestyle involves habitual behavior that is good for one's health. These determine what effects various seasons and places have on the individual body. We should keep harmony with the environment and stay connected with society. This book focuses on the impact of lifestyle on health from three aspects, adapting to the natural environment or climate, such as sunlight, air, and water, adjusting according to different life stages, and choosing or utilizing a suitable place to maintain health. Our surroundings affect our constitution, whether those influences are physical (such as weather, pollution, or seasonal changes) or social/emotional (friends, co-workers, and support systems). When we understand those elements, we can make the best choices for our lifestyle.

Healthy Rhythms and Rhythm Disorder-Related Illnesses

A healthy rhythm involves the body's internal biological clock marking days, months, seasons, and various life stages. The principle of the internal rhythms was proposed in 1959 by researcher Fianz Halberg at the Chronobiology Laboratory of the University of the Minnesota of the United States. He introduced the term daily rhythm, which refers to the internal rhythms of the body within a 24-hour period, including blood pressure, body temperature, sleep/

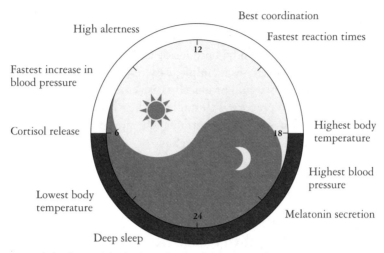

Internal rhythms of the body within a 24-hour period.

wake cycle, digestion, and neural sensitivity.

Daily prosody is one type of biological clocks. Prosody with less than 24 hours is called ultra-radian rhythms (heartbeat, breath rate), and prosody with a longer period is called infra-radian rhythms, such as monthly rhythms (female menstruation), circannual rhythms (fertility period, birth cycle, lifetime), and so on.

All life must adapt to the rotation of the earth. For many years, we have been aware that all living organisms, including humans, have an internal biological clock that allows them to adapt to day and night and find the rhythms of life. The work of Jeffrey C. Hall, Michael Rosbash, and Michael W. Young has tapped into the secret of the circadian clock, separating the genes that control the normal circadian rhythms of an organism and explaining how it works. Their research explains how plants, animals, and humans adapt to this biological rhythm and keep pace with the earth's rotation. The trio won the 2017 Nobel Prize in Physiology and Medicine for their work.

Our internal clocks provide very precise adjustments to our physiological functions at different times of the day, such as behavior, hormone levels, sleep, body temperature, and metabolism. When the external environment is mismatched with our body's clock, our physical condition will immediately reflect discomfort, such as the time difference caused by a flight across several time zones. There are also signs if our lifestyle begins to deviate from the body's biological clock, the risk of encountering various diseases will increase. This regular adaptation is called the circadian rhythm.

Our biological clocks allow our physiological mechanisms to predict and adapt to different times each day. The biological clock regulates some of the body's key functions, including blood pressure, eating, and sleeping rhythms. For example, at night, the pineal gland in the brain secretes increased levels of melatonin (Yin) and serotonin (Yin), which can help people sleep peacefully, but during the day, melatonin secretion is reduced and dopamine (Yang) secretion is enhanced, allowing people to work at full strength. Melatonin can also aid in dealing with jet lag, relieve stress, resolve mood disorders, and provide a strong antioxidant that neutralizes and scavenges free radicals. The secretion rhythm of melatonin is regarded as one of the body's biological clocks.

When our lifestyle deviates from our circadian clock, the risk of suffering from various diseases increases. The dysregulation of the biological clock can lead to insomnia, fatigue, depression, immune dysfunctions, and even various diseases, including tumors. For example, diabetes is found to be associated with the circadian clock. Epidemiological studies have found that workers who work across three shifts are more likely to develop Type II Diabetes than the average person. Researchers found that melatonin is associated with the onset of Type II Diabetes because of a variant in the gene associated with the hormone.

The study also found that the expression of the circadian clock gene in the brain of suicidal patients with severe depression differs significantly from that of ordinary people. The risk of tumors in rotation workers is related to the circadian clock disorder in tissues and organs. Heart attacks, asthma attacks, and arthritis pain all present a 24-hour rhythm, including the intestinal flora that is also regulated by the circadian clock. Of course, many of these processes are interactive.

Application of the Biological Clock through TCM
Since the three Nobel Prize winners made these pioneering discoveries, studies of circadian rhythms have evolved into a broad, highly active field of research. Through the study of the

biological clock, new disciplines such as time biology, chronology pharmacology, and time treatment have been introduced. It is evident that the study of the biological clock is of great significance in medicine and promotes basic theoretical biology research. For instance, I suggest that professional managers who travel frequently around the world take Ginkgo biloba pills or spleen and kidney Qi tonic pills because they cross multiple time zones, which can achieve or exceed the effects of melatonin, reduce the effects of jet lag and edema, and reduce the level of discomfort.

In TCM, each day is divided into four seasons. Early morning is spring, midday is summer (Yang), dusk is autumn, and late night is winter (Yin). In the *Yellow Emperor's Internal Canon of Medicine*, this theory is used to explain some diseases and emotional disorders. Morning tends to be a lighter time of release and rising, midday feels like a high point of peace, complaints and negative emotions arise at dusk, and the worst time is at night. Midnight is the point of deepest Yin and midday highest Yang. In Chinese medicine, 2 am is the turning point of Yang energy, when disease can turn either to death or recovery. If it is unable to turn, that means Yang cannot grow and overtake Yin. Four am is when Yang energy rises more rapidly. If it is unable to rise, it is a turning point. Early morning from 6 am to 9 or 10 am, our blood pressure and blood viscosity tend to be higher and there is less liquid in the body, so drinking water upon waking each morning is an important way to prevent cardiovascular and cerebrovascular diseases and prevent constipation. Yang energy rises like the sun, so a good breakfast encourages a healthy rise of Yang energy, since disorders and emotions are controlled by your physiological rise in energy. By midday, Yang energy rises to its pinnacle. A relaxing, rich, nutritional lunch is good for maintaining an orderly balance. Good energy at lunch can purge toxins and illness from the body, and one should consume carbohydrates, protein, and warm foods for lunch. The body has the capacity to feel its potential at this time. At dusk, the Yang energy starts to dissipate and Yin energy takes over. If dinner is consumed too late, it can be difficult to support energy toward the end of the day. A weakened body is then more susceptible to illness, disease, and emotional fluctuations. In the middle of the night, all of our Yang energy is hiding in the organs. It is a time of healing, and superficially, the body is weaker and more susceptible to outside factors and foreign elements. There is no energy to fight pathogenic elements and diseases can escalate to an unmanageable degree.

The *Yellow Emperor's Internal Canon of Medicine* also discusses the life processes of human growth, development, strengthening, and aging, along with the lifetime performance and physiological characteristics at different stages. The early growth period, transition time, and aging stage each need compensation and care.

A Daily Rhythm for Our Lives

TCM teaches that the best times to eat, sleep, work, and think are all set out like clockwork.

Meal rhythms: we should eat three meals a day in order to refresh Yang and Yin energies (breakfast between 7 and 9 am, lunch between 11 am and 1 pm, and dinner between 5 and 7 pm). Our daily energy starts flowing when we eat breakfast. It is best to have a warm breakfast that includes a good mix of various nutrients, like proteins, good fat, fiber, and carbohydrates.

You can have functional food for breakfast. A nutritious breakfast could include jujube 6 pieces, Chinese yam 15 g, walnut 2 pieces, dolichos seed 10 g, edible pine nut 10 g, and dry Chinese hawthorn 3 pieces. A balanced, nutritious lunch is important, though it does not have to be too heavy. Take a slow walk after lunch and massage the stomach and lower back to activate the spleen and kidneys. The best time for dinner is 2 to 3 hours before bedtime. The proportion of one's daily nutritional at dinnertime can be slightly smaller than breakfast and lunch. After dinner, do moderate exercise for 20 minutes to help digestion and absorption, encourage good sleep, and maintain your weight.

Study or work rhythms: the times between breakfast and lunch, lunch and dinner, and dinner and sleep are the best times for physical and mental activity.

Sleep rhythms: it is best to start deep sleep between 11 pm and midnight, then sleep well from 1 am to 5 am. Sleep is the best tool for cleansing the brain. After lunch, include 10 minutes of slow movements in your regimen, drink a little flower tea, and lie down and relax for 20 minutes.

Elimination rhythms: you should move the bowels between

5 am and 7 am "Don't let the old food meet new food" is an old saying in TCM.

Exercise rhythms: in spring and summer, we should get up earlier, so exercise should come before breakfast. In autumn and winter, we should get up later, so exercise will come in the afternoon before supper. It is best to drink something or eat a small portion of food before starting exercise.

Four Seasons of Health Care

In TCM theory, spring and summer are Yang seasons, while autumn and winter are Yin seasons. All Yin-Yang energy is influenced by the flow and change of seasons. Energy grows in the spring (*chun sheng*), reaching the highest level of the year in summer (*xia zhang*). Energy recedes in the autumn (*qiu shou*) and goes into quiet storage in the winter (*dong cang*). Cooking methods should follow the season, including steamed food in spring, raw food in summer, soup or sweet jelly in autumn, and stews or liquids from mixed foods in winter.

Although we may not realize it, our bodies automatically regulate our metabolism to adapt to seasonal changes. For example, if our bodies cannot properly warm up in the winter, we will feel cold, which may lead to a lack of energy. We need to assist and fine-tune our body's natural regulation system. One of the best and most natural ways to repair our system and maintain equilibrium is through the use of proper foods and herbs, as well as applying topical warming methods to meridians or stimulating the meridian points.

The "control system" of the body, like that in the home, relies on energy and a network of connections. The body's energy comes from the Blood and Qi. The blood vessels serve as a sort of visible cable network, while the meridians, which connect major organ systems, are invisible.

Spring, summer, autumn and winter are the seasons through which our mental and physical energy germinates, grows, strengthens, and ages. Childhood is similar to spring, which is always full of vitality, while youth is similar to summer, filled with growth and maturity. Middle age is autumn, a more introverted period of harvest, while old age is similar to winter, when one stores energy for the next cycle. The four seasons are similar to the rhythms of a day. The internal organs and their meridians have corresponding

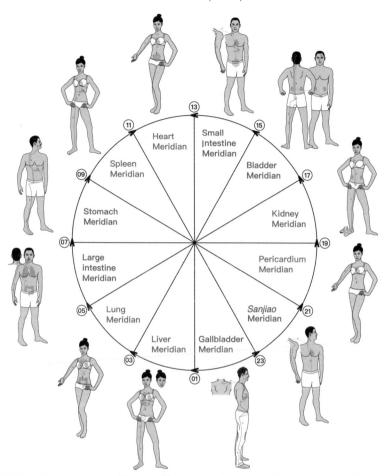

TCM 24-hour rhythm of internal organs and their meridians. Each meridian is most active in corresponding timeslot.

active periods at dawn, noon, dusk, and midnight, and the ups and downs are like summer and winter. The activities of one day should be consistent with the rising and store of Yang. Through the span of a lifetime, a year, or a day, the five internal *zang* organs and the six *fu* organs will only enjoy a smooth energy flow through a balanced opening and closing of the energy channels.

1. Spring

During the spring, all living things start to revive and grow. The plants and animals are resuscitated and flourish. Yang energy is rising and spreading, while Yin is decreasing. As the dominant mammal, humans should follow natural principles and take good care of ourselves, especially the liver.

Emotions: emotional stability is the capstone of a person's health. In the spring, people's emotions mimic the regeneration of other species like plants or animals after a winter's hibernation. Upon waking, their vitality is restored to its full level. Human emotions vary widely, as this quick jump into spring can induce many changes, such as feeling sleepy in the daytime, hay fever, facial skin rashes, and, especially, an increase in sex drive. It can also bring on recurring psychoses to their fullest degree. The body tends to go through a period in which rising energy levels need to be channeled. An inability to release the sex drive during this time causes emotional disorders and imbalances in the body.

Lifestyle: we should get up early in the morning in the spring to welcome the sun and take a walk outdoors to relax the body and enliven the mind. Compared with winter, we might sleep a bit later at night. It is often said that "spring weather changes three times a day, just like the smile on a child's face." Similarly, we are often told that "if we put on more clothes in the spring and wear less in the autumn, we will not be affected by various diseases." Putting on more clothes in spring is a traditional way to keep healthy in China, because the temperature in spring is uncertain, with warm air coming in as mother earth is still in need of a bit more time to warm up. We need to increase or decrease clothing in order to balance the body's temperature.

Diet and therapy: our body's spring metabolism has a certain connection with the liver, and like the seasonal changes, our energy's opening and rising is influenced by a rhythm. Spring is the season of germination, and the diet should be based on the principle of assisting the rise of Yang. One should eat Warm foods such as onions, ginger, garlic, alfalfa, and mustard, and consume less Cold food, such as melons and mung beans. If the temperature is high, it is necessary to prevent the Yang from rising too much. Otherwise, there will be stagnation and Heat. To prevent this, we should eat more light vegetables and sweet and sour fruits.

• Eat Warm food and take Sweet and slightly Acidic foods more frequently to maintain the balance of the liver and the digestive functions.

• Eat more yellow and green foods, such as fresh beans, peas, and wild vegetable sprouts so that the energy will rise and spread to the surface of the body.

• Moderately alter your protein and fat intake from that in the winter, consuming more eggs, milk, and nuts, and add plant proteins, dried or fresh beans, sprouts, and similar items. With the shortage of vitamins and minerals in the winter, it is necessary to introduce more seasonal wild vegetables to the kitchen during the spring, such as shepherd's purse (amaranth), portulaca oleracea L., dandelion, plantain, sprouts of Kalimeris indica (L.), or spring bamboo shoots, to maintain the needs of the body in order to prevent flu, spring dermatitis, and canker sores.

2. Summer

From June to August, natural plants have blossomed and are at their richest. Summer is a time of rising heat, and because the metabolism increases, most will sweat more during these months. It is important to follow natural principles to take care of yourself, especially the heart and brain functions.

Emotions: summer emotions are more Yang in nature, and thus more outwardly expressive. During this time of the year, people are more extroverted and generally happier and more enthusiastic. However, a lack of sleep and humid weather can lead people to feel annoyed and agitated. Those with a warmer constitution who like to eat red meat might tend to become more irritable and angrier if they have too much Yang in the system.

Lifestyle: summer's cultivation of health follows the sunrise and sunset, sleeping a bit later and getting up earlier, with some rest in the middle of the day to prevent one from feeling too hot, which puts strain on the heart system. Eat more Cool nourishing foods to keep the Summer-Heat from disturbing your health. The heart Qi is strongest in summer, which might dominate the body's Spirit. *The Yellow Emperor's Internal Canon of Medicine* states that "the heart is the king of body's activities," and if the heart Qi is abundant, we will feel refreshed. Therefore, people born in this season are often extroverted, lively, active, and communicative. If the heart Qi is not balanced with Body Fluid and Blood, it can turn to heart Heat. Heart Heat can easily lead to diseases such as skin sores or sunstroke, or if one uses heart energy excessively in the summer, the heart Qi can weaken, which may lead to dizziness, chest pressure, shortness of breath, or the early stages of cardiovascular diseases.

Diet and therapy: according to the characteristics of summer, Yang energy is most vigorous at this time, so health care in the summer should pay attention to the growth of Yang, not to consuming too much iced and cold food.

Summertime is when all natural plants bloom and are most exposed. It is the moment when nature is rapidly growing and flowering, showing its prosperity. This is also the best time to detoxify, cultivating Yang oxygen to treat winter diseases. This principle for cultivating health is called "treat winter issues in summer."

The period from the Summer Solstice (*xia zhi*) to the Beginning of the Autumn (*li qiu*) is called in the Southern part of China *san fu tian* (meaning the hottest days). People who are usually weaker in Yang will eat Hot foods, such as angelica ginger mutton soup. Skin issues can be treated with Gua Sha scraping or cupping, letting the toxic Heat discharge from the body with the opening of sweat pores. If you have respiratory issues, such as an asthmatic cough, sinuses in the winter, or sore joints, you can also improve it by applying moxibustion and herbal paste to the surface of the meridian points.

Since there are high temperatures and Dampness in summer, it is important to pay attention to the digestive system, using cooling foods to quell the Heat and bitter foods to remove the Dampness. One's diet should be Sweet and Cool, with some Bitter foods, such as mung bean soup, sprouts, watermelon, pearl barley, tofu, alfalfa, pumpkin, or bitter gourd, and less greasy or heavy foods.

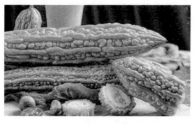

Enjoying some bitter foods in summer can clear the mind and eliminate restlessness, such as bitter gourd.

Enjoying some Bitter foods such as asparagus or green tea in the summer can not only clear the mind and eliminate restlessness, refreshing and sharpening the mental activity, but will also increase the appetite and harmonize gastrointestinal functions.

• It is advisable to eat more

yellow and red foods and raw foods, and frequently include a small quantity of Bitter foods.

• Eat more vegetables and gourds, such as watermelon, sweet melon, or towel gourd, to address the needs for Body Fluid and energy, since one is likely to experience heavy perspiration and a lack of sleep.

• Easily digestible and cooked (prepared) proteins like fresh roots, berries, mushrooms, or radishes, should be slightly decreased in summer for the sake of the digestive function.

3. Autumn

In early autumn, the weather goes back to a cooling state in which the wind blows, the sky is clear, the atmosphere becomes drier, and the leaves change color. Everything is ripening and ready for harvest. Compared with spring, the Yang energy gradually pulls back, declines, and shrinks, while Yin increases. The dry air can affect people prone to dehydration, especially in their lungs.

Emotions: this is usually a very soothing, enjoyable, relaxing time of year. However, as the season progresses, the cool air turns into a colder wind, the leaves wither and fall from the trees, and the days become noticeably shorter with gloomy skies. People suffer more pain in the body and joints. Emotions are in a repressed state and people are less expressive in public.

Lifestyle: as the Yang is adducted, people will prefer to go to bed a bit earlier than in summer and get up earlier than in winter. It is important to pay attention to the maintenance of Yang energy in the body. The Spirit, daily life, diet, and exercises should follow the principle of the autumn harvest. Moderate exposure to cold may induce our resistance to cold as we prepare for the coming winter. One will easily sweat if they put on thick clothing too early in the season, which does not match the principle of heath cultivation in autumn, which is to nourish Dryness.

Diet and therapy: in autumn, it is advisable to eat more nourishing foods. The lungs correspond to autumn. Sudden or excessive Coldness and Dryness can easily hurt the lung and cause one to catch the flu, a cough, bronchial asthma, and other respiratory diseases. Intensifying and moistening the lungs can help to prevent dry scalp, hair loss, and thirst. Eat more vegetables and fruits rich in fluids and include sesame, walnut, pear, fresh jujube,

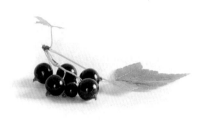

Blackcurrants.

chrysanthemum tea, and white fungus in your diet, but eat less spicy and sweat inducing foods.

In the fall, the lungs are most vulnerable to external attack. Children and the elderly require extra care. Almonds, ginkgo nuts, lily bulbs, and lotus seeds contain good nutrition for lung function.

• Consume moistening and nourishing foods, with some seeds and nuts. If you often sweat and pass soft stool, add some sweet and sour berries like blackcurrants or schisandra berries.

• Eat more food containing jelly, like white fungus, flaxseed, sticky rice, and gluey millet.

• Eat more orange and white foods, like fresh fruits and herbal roots juices like pear, water chestnut, lotus root, and radix polygonati officinalis.

4. **Winter**

When winter comes, the weather reaches its greatest extreme in cold. Everything freezes, the earth cracks, and some plants and animals go into hibernation, which is similar to humans' physical and mental functions. The cold air can affect those who lack energy, especially in the kidney organ. One's daily routine will conform to the needs of the body to replenish and strengthen the Yang.

Emotions: your own ambitions are less exposed in winter. The coldest season is a private moment for self-care and to be more self-conscious. This is the time to engage in self-satisfaction and self-enjoyment, and also the best time for you to sit and meditate or practice Qigong, as you are quiet on the inside. In addition, for some of us, emotions may stagnate. It can become easy to look at life in a more negative way, and those negative thoughts may come into our dreams or suddenly appear in our mind. If we follow the principle of "autumn and winter nourish Yin" and "reinforce the kidney and prevent Cold," while "not disturbing Yang," we can moderate our emotions.

Lifestyle: we should pay attention to protecting Yang, recharging our batteries for the next year. Try not to sweat too much or eat raw, iced, and cold foods that disturb the Yang. Sleep earlier and get up later, in order to avoid the early morning frost and wait for sunrise before going out in the morning. The only season in which one should sleep longer and get up later is winter. In winter, the day is shorter and the night is longer, so daylight hours are the shortest of any other season in the year. Try not to go barefoot or expose the belly. In winter, the energy and Blood functions are weak between the head and neck. The three acupoints in this area are called Fengchi (GB 20), Fengfu (GV 16), and Yifeng (TE 17), and they are the most vulnerable areas to Coldness and Wind, so the neck should be protected. It is necessary to keep indoor temperatures in a stable range and to pay attention to spending more time in the sun, because the sun can warm up and strengthen the human body, help blood circulation, and gives us the ability to protect ourselves from winter viruses. We must likewise pay attention to protection from Coldness and Wind, wearing thick, soft, warm clothing. Select darker clothing, wear cotton underwear, loose outerwear, shoes, and socks, and keep the hands, feet, and ears warm. If we don't store kidney energy in the winter, we will lose our Essence. Like a perennial plant, there will be no motivation and no nutrients in the next spring.

Diet and therapy: the kidneys correspond to winter. The digestive function is active, so especially strengthening the kidneys and related organs should be a priority. It is often said that we should "supplement in winter, then there will be no disease in the coming year," pointing to a popular method of prevention. In Shanghai in mid and late November, many clients come to the Chinese medicine hospital or clinic and ask for a consultation. After the consultation, the doctor gives them 5 to 7 days of herbal decoctions for regular energy movement and blood circulation and harmony in the digestive functions. At the same time, they will prescript an herbal paste similar to a fruit jelly. Clients will start taking this from the Winter Solstice, and continue throughout the winter until the following spring. By doing so, one can prevent and treat many recurring illnesses such as asthma, frostbite, winter flu, and sinusitis.

Diet is also based on harmonizing Yin and Yang. In winter, foods and tonics that protect against Coldness are often valued. To

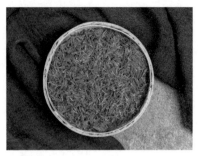

Saffron.

increase Yang, eat Warm foods such as lamb, oysters, raspberries, leeks, dried longan, jujubes, yams, walnuts, chestnuts, pine nuts, or peanuts. To warm the kidneys or harmonize Yin and Yang, you can eat cinnamon, rosemary, mustard seed, nutmeg, goji berries, saffron, and reishi mushroom. Eat various nuts with Warm or Hot temperatures and Spicy or Salty tastes, along with more yellow and black foods, such as brown and black rice, black kidney beans, black fungus, and black sesame seeds.

Following the daily and yearly rhythms and doing everything in moderate and balanced fashion are important aspects of prolonging life. It is a good habit to tone the organs before the season. In this way, Chinese people plan their diet a season in advance and take special care to include foods that help to balance the effects of the coming season. Since the digestive system is more active during winter, your body can digest food more effectively during these months. Since people are less active in winter and sleep longer, the nourishment consumed is easily stored as Essence instead of being spent. In saying this, however, it is always important to heed to the demands of your individual constitution.

Three Pre-Disease Stages

TCM focuses on preventative methods and taking action before illness or disease occurs. In order to be healthy, we need to be proactive and understand our energy, Blood, meridian movements, and immune system. There are typically three stages that occur prior to disease.

1. Healthy Phase: Focus on Prevention and Strengthening of Qi

We are generally in good health and should take measures to achieve balance and extend our lifespan. To do so, we must first know whether we have enough healthy Qi, then learn how to maintain or strengthen it. If we have healthy Qi, we can fight viruses and bacteria when others are getting sick, have a speedy recovery when we get injured, and our Blood and Qi will go to relevant areas of the body when needed without difficulty. For example, when you want to do work which requires concentration, your brain will have energy, and if you want to go running, the energy goes to your legs. It must be noted that jet lag can decrease healthy Qi because of time-zone differences and differences in one's routine.

In order to protect your Qi and prevent disease, it is important to avoid strong external environmental factors. To stay safe from viruses, you should protect yourself and avoid crowds at these times. If air pollution levels are high, make sure to use an air purifier, wear a mask, and avoid exercising outside. Bacteria and food contamination can also cause illness, so be vigilant with proper cooking and cleaning.

To utilize Qi most effectively, we must take life phases into consideration. Young adults, middle-aged adults, and seniors require different lifestyles and levels of energy. Failure to identify one's life phase will deplete Qi, and they will become sick easily.

2. Early Onset: Recognize Symptoms and Take Action to Improve Health

Clinical symptoms such as running nose, cough, insomnia, or a lack of energy lead us to take action. With these early onset symptoms, we can take a self-help approach and perhaps not need to see a medical professional at all. This approach can be carried out at home and addressed through diet.

Those who are intolerant to Coldness and have an increased chance of catching colds in winter should consume soup, water, and ginger tea, add onions and garlic to food, eat plenty of fruits, rest, and conserve energy to fight the illness.

For a fever or sore throat, which is typically intolerant to Summer-Heat, add mint, lemon, honey, chrysanthemum, watermelon juice, cucumber juice, and pear juice to the diet and apply a cold compress to the forehead.

There are a number of ways to identify early onset symptoms, as external signs can often indicate internal changes. According to the *Yellow Emperor's Internal Canon of Medicine*, there are 4 methods of diagnosis using the sense organs. We can use seeing, listening, smelling, and feeling to identify changes to the normal state before seeking medical advice.

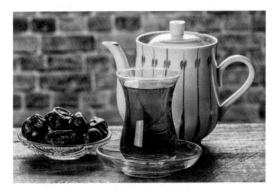

Jujube tea.

Seeing: changes in face color and puffy or dull eyes, tongue coating changes from thin to thick or from white to gray or yellow.

Listening: hoarse or low voice, sneezing, or heavy breathing.

Smelling: smell in the mouth, or excretions from our body like sweat, urine, or stool become strange in smell.

Feeling: skin, muscles, nails, meridian sensitivity, and nodules.

There is currently a global novel Coronavirus pandemic caused by a flu. Some people contracted the virus then recovered within 10 to 14 days. In others, the disease developed rapidly, then led to organ failure. When analyzing cases using the principles of TCM, there will be differences in the treatment of early symptoms, which is determined by the different constitutions of the patients and early responses to the disease.

Neck stiffness from stress or excessive exercise can be treated with warm patches on the local area for 2 hours and drinking jujube tea. Acute kidney and liver infection will show signals on the surface of the body. For instance, Hepatitis A leads to yellow eyes, skin, and urine. Acute kidney issues will change the texture (turbid and foam), color (brown, white, red), and quantity of urine. Chronic diarrhea with weight loss can be due to stomach or colon issues. It is essential to take note of changes in urine and stool. If urine contains bubbles or becomes foggy, it is an indication that the kidneys cannot retain protein. If the urine contains bubbles and has a sweet smell, it is important to check the blood sugar. Tumors, stones, and cysts are difficult to identify from the outside, so it is necessary to conduct tests and an ultrasound scan to determine the causes.

3. Sickness or Disease: If Symptoms Worsen, Seek

Professional Medical Advice

We may experience early onset of a disease in which symptoms escalate and cannot be treated at home. These can be acute or chronic and will require us to see a doctor. Examples include acid reflux, duodenal ulcer, diarrhea, sinus problems, influenza, common cold, pain, and irregular menstruation.

With the escalation of a sore throat to a cough, it is important to see a doctor if there is no improvement after 3 days. In some cases, it can develop into an infection, and in very old or young people, it can progress into pneumonia. In Western medicine, antibiotics and antivirals are used to tackle the illness. In TCM, patterns (Cold/ Hot/Dry/Damp/weak) are identified so you can take action at home to speed up recovery and prevent a relapse. Though often effective, medicine alone is not always enough. For a prompt, effective recovery, we need to pair antibiotics with food, drink, and herbs to address body patterns and ensure you build up healthy Qi. Using diet alongside medicine can stop virus or bacteria from spreading from one part of the body to a secondary organ, such as a throat infection moving to the heart, which becomes difficult to fight because the immune system is already weak, or from the lung to colon and causing colitis, which requires additional treatment.

For cancer patients, surgery, radiotherapy, or chemotherapy is often required to eliminate the cancer. These procedures are extremely harmful and invasive to a healthy body. TCM can play a complementary role in treating cancer, helping to limit the condition's spread through the body and ensuring higher levels of healthy Qi.

Before surgery, herbal remedies can be used to build up healthy Qi, usually for around 3 months. During treatment, continue to use food therapy, acupuncture, and warm methods to maintain healthy Qi levels, usually for 2 to 5 years. After treatment, regulate and tone organs and keep Qi, Blood, and Body Fluid levels high through diet and lifestyle regulation for at least 6 months.

In ancient times, only herbal remedies were used, as there were no antibiotics, steroids, or other modern medicines. In modern times, we use a combination of holistic strategy (TCM) and local precision (modern) medicine for health care.

Western medicine, or white box theory, is based on anatomy.

White box theory primarily uses cause and effect to identify and treat illness. The methods and treatments are developed clinical or through laboratory studies. Taking Alzheimer's disease as an example, modern medicine states that one reason people suffer from Alzheimer's disease is that when cerebrovascular disease hardens the artery, the quantity of blood reaching to the brain is reduced, causing the brain to shrink. The focus of TCM is more holistic, collecting all external and internal information on the body, using the five organ system to identify the patterns of the liver, kidneys, heart, lungs, and spleen before treating this disease. For Alzheimer's, TCM identifies the problem early on through patterns with heart blood stagnation and with kidney Essence shortages. The symptoms are a lack of sleep, poor memory, frequent urination, and lower back pain. Herbal remedies, acupuncture, and massage can be used to address regular blood circulation and open the capillaries to delay the progress of Alzheimer's.

Life Cultivation Based on Life Stages

Confucius (551–479 BC), the father of Confucianism in the Spring and Autumn and the Warring States, has many incisive opinions on health preservation and longevity. He divided human life into three stages according to the physiological and psychological situation. There are some precautions to be avoided of each stage. For example, too many temptations should be avoided in adolescence, because at this time our bodies are not yet mature. In middle age, avoid excessive mental competitiveness. Don't always think that you are outstanding or superior, a kind of character flaw that easily occurs in our most vigorous stage. At this time, people have lofty aspirations and feel that they can achieve anything they want, but if they exceed their physiological and psychological tolerance, they will plant the seeds of cardiovascular and cerebrovascular diseases. In old age, we should avoid excessive temperance and greed, because at this period, our energy is insufficient. Excessive effort and insatiability will bring greater wear and tear to the body.

In different periods of life, we should use a rational approach to restrain the wild horse of emotions and desire, so as to achieve cohesiveness and moderation.

According to the different stages of the human life cycle, there

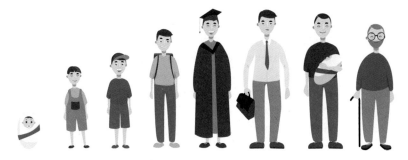

There are different requirements for the diet, emotions, and mental care for different stages of the human life.

are different requirements for the diet, emotions, and mental care.

1. Childhood

It is said that "if you want your child to be safe, leave them three percent hungry and cold." It means that children should not wear anything too warm or eat too full because they are young and the function of viscera is not yet mature, while the vitality of children grows strong and Yang energy goes upward. Dietary nutrition needs to be comprehensive and balanced, but food intake cannot be too great or it will be difficult to digest and absorb, which may cause other diseases. Excessive intake of rich foods or dietary supplements will lead to the early development of the reproductive endocrine system and precocious puberty. Also, because a child has more vitality and Yang energy, they should not wear too much clothes to prevent excessive perspiration. Frequent sweating and open pores, especially in autumn and winter, will lead to colds and cause viral diseases. In addition, the health care of children and adolescents should focus on whether the physiological and psychological indicators of each stage are aligned. Parents can consciously cultivate their children's concept of disease prevention. For example, from the moment a child is born, a health record is established for them. It includes birth conditions, family history, and childhood medical history, as well as their growth and development and psychological status in various periods. By the time the child turns 18 and goes to college, it is recommended you give this health file to the child as their rite of passage. The children continue to write their own life and health records after the age of 18.

2. Young Adults

With the increasing burden of learning and facing the choices of school, friends, family, career, and other major life decisions, the health care of young adults should focus on emotional and mental health. Each of us should be aware of our emotional type, our ability to cope with stress, and how to use the resources of our support system. Emotions are the keys to long-term health. Both the body and mind or internal organs and soul need to be cared for and nourished. The body needs to be active, and the mind needs to be calm. These days, there are many things that influence us from the outside and disturb the mind. We are now living in a world where people are increasingly distracted and constantly experience high levels of stress. It is essential to find methods to keep our mental focus and create balance with our physical body. Incorporate methods that help calm the mind and bring clarity and focus. Most importantly, find time to do something you like to do. It sounds simple, but people often neglect their own passions or hobbies because of the fast pace and stress of life. Finding time to do something that relaxes you should not be overlooked.

Both men and women have their own characteristics. The physiological peak for a woman is between 32 to 35 years old, while for a man it is between 36 and 40 years old. After that, it remains stable for quite a long time, then gradually declines. If we pay proper attention to maintaining Qi and Blood and regulate the functions of our liver and digestive systems before and after the peak period, we can lay a better foundation for later life.

3. Senior Period

When women are around 55 and men are around 65, the physiological functions tend to decay, including pre-menopause or menopausal symptoms. In some cases, we may experience impaired digestive functions, mental fatigue, decreased attention and memory, shorter sleep times, and decreased vision and hearing. Hair grays, and body shape changes. We call it deficiency in both the spleen and kidneys and a lack of energy and Blood. The protection of the spleen and stomach, the maintaining of the digestive system functions, the increase of kidney energy, and the practice of Qigong exercise are the primary tasks in senior health care. Specifically, we should take good care of ourselves after retirement. The arrival of menopause and the process of entering retirement is not only a transition stage, but also life's second spring. This is when children grow up and leave home, and the intensity of work decreases significantly. We have enough time to choose a new career or hobby. How do we adjust our interests and rhythm of life? How do we smoothly transit from career-centered work to life based on one's interest? From my contact with a large number of healthy people with long lives, the life of healthy seniors can be summarized as follows:

First, welcome the arrival of the senior years with a calm, optimistic attitude. Although we have various symptoms of aging, it is like a plant going from youth to strength, then to decline, which is a natural evolutionary process, so accept it calmly and do not worry too much.

Second, pay more attention to yourself, your family, and to social events. Develop one or two new hobbies and broaden your circle of friends, constantly interacting with them to deepen mutual understanding. Build deep friendships. Talk with people and keep good connections with society. In ancient times, talking was a good way to move our body energy and speed up mental activity when there weren't as many different forms of exercise available. People need to talk and express themselves in order to be healthy. The main reason women have higher rates of depression is that they often lack the opportunity to fully express themselves or talk enough. Talking or singing to yourself is a great way to maintain health. After talking and expressing ourselves, worries, anxieties, and depression can be managed and eliminated. Many people believe eating foods can help with detoxing, but actually talking helps too. It is a good way to maintain mental and emotional health.

Third, adjust the rhythm of your life and diet to a more regular and suitable track for our own constitution. Ensure that you have adequate sleep and a good appetite, and pay attention to moderate cleansing of the body's metabolites through sweating, especially during spring and summer, and smooth and regular urine and stool. Take two to three kinds of plant-based foods, for instance ginseng and schisandra berries which offers dual regulation of blood sugar, blood pressure, and immune system functions. Select three to five body surface acupoints to regulate the circulation of Qi and Blood in the limbs and joints, and ensure adequate nutrition for your muscles and skin, such as the Zusanli point (ST 36), Baihui point (GV 20), Guanyuan point (CV 4), and Qihai point (CV 6).

Ecosystem, Geographical Regions, and Health

Our physical and emotional states are greatly influenced by climate, the environment, and its rhythm and seasons. The geographical features of a place have a strong impact on both our body constitution and our food choices. People from the north can tolerate hotter foods than those who have grown up in the south. People from humid regions can tolerate wet climates better than people from dry regions. For instance, if you live in an area that is very dry, you might do something to counteract it and balance the Dryness, like consuming more goji berries. In China, people eat a lot

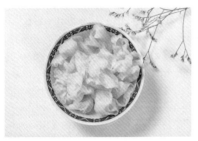

Tremella or white fungus.

of lily bulbs (in food and drink), tremella, pears, and avocados in autumn and winter to counteract the Dryness of the environment during that time. These foods nourish the lungs and protect them from Dryness. In Beijing, they might consume these foods a little more often than those living in Shanghai, due to the fact that Beijing is drier.

1. Regional Advantages

Regional health care depends on geographical environment characteristics, because constitutions and food choices of people from different regions vary. The unique features of a local environment always give its inhabitants special characteristics.

People from the north can take more Hot foods and herbs. For example, in the northwest and northeast of China, where the climate is cold and the air is dry, people eat more beef and mutton and less vegetables and fruits, and they favor stronger tastes. Their cooking methods are mostly roasting, frying, and grilling. A meat diet has higher calories and helps protect them from the Coldness. When they suffer from Cold types of illnesses, they can tolerate a higher dosage of warming herbs than people from southern areas.

However, people living in humid areas prefer to consume foods that remove Dampness or induce diuresis. There are accumulated experiences in regional diet therapies for those living in the mountain areas of Chongqing or living along the seaside of Guangdong. In both areas, local people are more likely to have symptoms of Dampness. The climate in Sichuan and Hunan provinces is chilling and damp, so it is not surprising that Sichuan and Hunan cuisines are famous for their dried spices. These spices can be applied to overcome Dampness and Cold symptoms. Guangdong has a hot climate and is dominated by Damp Heat. In order to resist hot, humid disturbances, residents are used to apply cooling herbal teas and soups, including barley or lentils, to remove Dampness and induce diuresis.

Some areas are havens for health. *The Yellow Emperor's Internal Canon of Medicine* points out that a quieter ecosystem helps people balance themselves. Doctors Sun Simiao in the Tang dynasty and Gong Yanxian from the Ming dynasty emphasized that a cool mountain climate with fresh air and sunshine allows people to enjoy themselves and promotes their metabolism, enhancing the body's resistance to diseases. It has been proven to be a holy area for health cultivation.

The mineral springs of Wudalianchi City, located in Heihe City, Heilongjiang Province, is one of the world's three major cold springs (the other two are the French Vichy mineral springs and the Russian North Caucasus mineral springs). Cold spring water contains high concentrations of soda and some metasilicic acid, and it is slightly alkaline. Drinking spring water allows the residents to keep fit and treat illness. The spring can also be utilized in topical bathing to achieve soft, shiny, elastic skin and to treat skin issues.

The volcanic group in the Wudalianchi area is 400 to 600 meters above sea level. It is famous for its special structure of volcanic cones, various volcanic lava flow patterns, lava tunnels filled with frost, and cold carbonated mineral springs. The Wudalianchi volcanic slime has gradually formed over 300,000 years and contains more than 60 kinds of beneficial elements such as calcium, magnesium, potassium, silicon, iron, sulfur, and special minerals, which are excellent for both medical and health care. Glacial muds, dead sea mud, and volcanic slime can make our skin and body healthier, and the combination of cold springs and volcanic slime is most unique here.

Magnetic therapy (magneto therapy) is a method for treating

certain diseases by applying natural or artificial magnetic fields to the human meridians, acupoints, and local area of illness. According to the research, it is believed that magnetic fields can regulate the biological magnetic field in human body, generate induced micro-currents, change the permeability of cell membranes, regulate the activity of certain enzymes, expand blood vessels, and accelerate blood flow, achieving ancillary effects such as pain relief and reduced swelling.

Reports show that magnetic therapy is effective for hypertension, arthritis, headaches, insomnia, coronary heart disease, gastroenteritis, facial muscle spasms, sprains, and cervical spondylosis. Attention should be given to the concentration of the magnetic field. Less concentration of the magnetic field may not achieve a desired therapeutic effect, while too high a concentration of the magnetic field may have side effects on the human body, such as dizziness and vomiting, among others.

In summer, the Wudalianchi pool gathers the volcano, geomagnetism, hot springs, cold spring water, and sunlight in one place, becoming a magical health paradise. It has significant curative effects on various chronic diseases and geriatric diseases such as neck, waist and leg ailments, oral diseases, varicose veins, and postpartum issues.

Therapies involving drinking spring water and using it to wash the body have been among the local people for thousands of years, and have a magical effect on rehabilitation and recuperation and for health and longevity.

2. Regional Disadvantages

Modern medical research has found that in addition to climate, sun, air, and season, other factors such as local land resources, including various trace elements, pollution of water and drinking water, and vegetation damage, can also have an impact on the human body. It has been confirmed that some of the endemic diseases are often related to a lack or an excess of certain trace elements in the local soil or water system. These are the adverse effects of the regional environment on the human body. Protecting yourself against these factors is the concern of regional health care. Natural environmental influences also impact the water and food that we intake. A healthy environment can help protect your body.

The ecosystem determines many common local illnesses. TCM teaches that all the flavors and colors of foods are mainly related to the soil. Keshan disease, also known as endemic cardiomyopathy, occurs in Keshan County, Heilongjiang Province of China. It is understood that it is due to a selenium deficiency. Endemic goiter is more common in inland mountainous areas that are far from the sea. It has a certain relationship with iodine deficiencies.

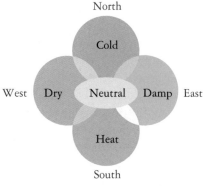

The relationship between ecology, climate, and individual types.

The ecosystem leads to different types of illnesses. The types of arthritis in the wet areas south of the Yangtze River is mostly caused by Heat and Dampness. Arthritis in northwestern China is mostly caused by Wind and Coldness.

People living in the areas close to nuclear radiation and nuclear pollution sites inevitably see a dramatic increase in cancer rates.

3. TCM Foods and Acupoints to Overcome Regional Health Issues

Food and acupressure can help you overcome regional issues. When considering locality and season, we face some simple and some complicated conditions. For instance, summer is longer in the southern regions, and thus more Heat disturbs the local residents, while those who live in the southeast or live in the coastal areas are more likely to combine Heat and Dampness. Here, we will provide some advice for those with Damp (Dry) and Heat (Cold) constitutions for dealing with complex symptoms.

• People living in temperate zones or those with Neutral individual types can follow their life stages, the growth, strengthening and aging stages. People in both the growth and aging stages need more nutrition. They will obtain nutrition from beans, seeds, nuts, and roots, such as olives, sunflower seeds, carrots, malt, black beans, peanuts, grapes, and pumpkins. They can massage, tap, or perform Gua Sha on the Heart, Spleen, and Kidney Meridians points, such as the Shenmen (HT 7), Baihui (GV 20),

Zusanli (ST 36), and Taixi (KI 3) points.

• People living in the southwest regions or with Dry and Hot individual types with symptoms such as itchy scalp and dandruff, dry skin, and frequent feelings of heat and thirst should consume more apples, asparagus, lily bulbs, millet, wheat, citrus fruits, oysters, and straw mushrooms. They should use Yin meridian points such as the Taichong (LR 3), Sanyinjiao (SP 6), and Guanyuan (CV 4) points.

• People living in the southeast regions or with Damp and Hot individual types who feel hot and heavy, with increased secretions from the nose and/or eyes, or who feel sticky and need to clear their throats regularly can consider consuming celery, green tea, pearl barley, radish, dolichos seed, cooling tea, plantains, winter melon skin and seeds, dandelion root, marine algae, and selfheal (spica prunellae vulgaris L.). They should use the Large Intestine and Spleen Meridian points such as the Quchi (LI 4), Hegu (LI 11), and Yinlingquan (SP 9) points.

• For people living in the northwest areas or who have Cold with Dryness individual types, symptoms might include aversion to Coldness, thirst, a preference for warmer water or drinks, numbness and tendon spasms, and a preference for warmer areas. They should consume angelica roots, chicken, chives (leek seed), raspberries, pine nuts, glutinous rice, longan, walnuts, and schisandra berries. They should use the Gallbladder and Bladder Meridian points such as the Shenshu (BL 23), Jingmen (GB 25), snd Xuanzhong (GB 39).

• People living in the northeast areas or who have Cold and Damp individual types might feel chest and abdominal bloating and experience full, lose bowel movements. They have low tolerance for cold drinks and iced water, edema in their limbs, and chills, and sometimes cough thin sputum. They should consume pepper (black or white), turmeric, capsicum, (chili peppers, cayenne, nutmeg, mustard seeds, rosemary, basil, cinnamon bark, cloves, and osmanthus. They should use the Governing Vessel and Conception Vessel and acupoints such as the Dazhui (GV 14) and Shuifen (CV 9) points, combined with moxibustion on local areas of discomfort.

Appendices

Basic Concepts of TCM Health Care Defined by the State Administration of Traditional Chinese Medicine

1. Traditional Chinese medicine health care refers to health activities guided by TCM theory to achieve physical fitness, prevent disease, and prolong life through various methods.

2. The concept of TCM health is to conform to nature, balance between Yin and Yang, and adapt to the individual.

3. Emotion, diet, lifestyle, and exercise are the four cornerstones of TCM health.

4. TCM health care emphasizes comprehensive maintenance and conditioning, starting from youth and lasting throughout one's entire life.

State Administration of Traditional Chinese Medicine
National Health and Family Planning Commission

May 16, 2014

Glossary

Blood: Blood is one of the essential substances that make up the human body and maintain the activities of life. It is a nutritious red fluid that flows in the vessels.

Blood is the mother of Qi: This idea refers to the influence of Blood on Qi, i.e. Blood conveys and nourishes Qi.

Body Fluid: Body Fluid is a general term for all the normal liquids in the body. It is one of the essential substances making up the human body and maintaining the activities of life.

Body Fluid and Blood share the same sources: Both Body Fluid and Blood are derived from the nutrients we absorb from food. Body Fluid is a component of Blood. Body Fluid and Blood can transform into each other in the body, so it is said that "Body Fluid and Blood share the same source."

Chest Qi (*zong qi*): Chest Qi is derived mainly from oxygen inhaled during exercise and from food essence. It is predominately stored in the Danzhong point (CV 17) between the lung and heart. Chest Qi keeps the airways open for the lungs. If it can effectively flow to the throat, singing and talking for long periods of time can be done easily and without discomfort. Chest Qi helps to warm the heart and promotes efficient blood circulation.

congenital base of life (congenital foundation): The body's constitution determined before birth is controlled by the kidneys and their function.

congenital natural disposition (endowment gift): Besides the kidneys, prenatal influences on the constitution include the state of nutrition and other influences on development. The health of a mother during pregnancy has an effect on the constitution.

constitution: Body constitution is formed before birth but can be influenced by factors after birth. The constitution comprises features of the body's structure and its physiological and psychological functions.

Defensive Qi (*wei qi*): It is produced mainly from the nutrients we absorb from food. The function of Defensive Qi is to protect the body against viruses, bacteria, Cold, or anything that may cause it harm. Defensive Qi is diffused under the skin. During the day, Defensive Qi surrounds the blood veins and meridians. At night, it moves into the organs. The lungs regulate its movement under the skin.

Essence (*jing*): Essence is one of the most valuable components of the human body, and consists of two aspects. The first refers to the basic material that forms the viscera, tissues, skin, hair, tendons, and muscles. The second refers to the reproductive Essence, which comprises not only the individual's own reproductive Essence but also the hereditary reproductive Essence (i.e. that of the parents). It is like a bridge between past generations and generations to come. The kidneys preserve and store Essence.

meridians and collaterals: Meridians and collaterals are pathways through which Qi and Blood circulate and through which the viscera and limbs are connected. They allow communication between the upper and lower parts and the interior and exterior parts of the body.

Nutrition Qi (*ying qi*): Nutrition Qi originates from nutrition in food, which is transformed by the spleen and stomach. It is a component part in the blood flowing throughout the body. Nutrition Qi circulates in the blood vessels and is transformed into blood to nourish the whole body.

Original Qi (*yuan qi*): Original Qi originates from congenital Essence, also known as kidney Qi. It is replenished and "topped up" by one's nutrition after birth. However, it declines as one begins to age.

Qi: It is the most fundamental substance of the human body. It is the energy or life-process that flows in and around all of us.

Qi is the commander of Blood: This idea emphasizes the influence of Qi on Blood. This influence covers three aspects, promoting blood production, blood circulation, and controlling Blood.

Qi transformation: The various changes associated with movements of Qi are called "Qi transformation."

source of acquired constitution: While the kidney is the congenital foundation of the constitution, the spleen is the source of the acquired constitution. The spleen system directs food transportation and transformation, playing a role in the digestion and assimilation of nutrients. These functions play an important role in the formation of Qi and Blood.

Spirit: In TCM theory, the term "Spirit" is an abstract concept. In the broad sense, it encompasses the outward activities of life and refers to the comprehensive whole. This includes the vitality of the body, appearance, complexion, expression of the eyes, speech, and responsiveness. In a narrow sense, Spirit is a collective term for cognition, consciousness, and other mental activities.

the eight extraordinary vessels: The name of the eight extraordinary vessels are *du mai* (the Governing Vessel), *ren mai* (the Conception Vessel), *chong mai* (the Thoroughfare Vessel), *dai mai* (the Belt Vessel), *yin qiao* (the Yin-Heel Vessel), *yang qiao* (the Yang-Heel Vessel), *yin wei* (the Yin-Link Vessel), and *yang wei* (the Yang-Link Vessel). The eight extraordinary vessels are different from the twelve regular meridians. The eight extraordinary vessels have no regular distribution, no direct connection with the viscera, and no internal and external relationship between each other.

the heart controls Blood and blood vessels: The heart governs the Blood and blood vessels of the body. All the blood and vessels of the body are subordinate to the heart. The heart Qi is the motive force for blood circulation and propels the blood to flow in the vessels, thereby maintaining the supply of nourishment to the whole body.

the heart houses the Spirit: This idea mainly refers to the supreme dominating factor of life activities throughout the body. It includes mental activities, consciousness, thinking, and sleeping. The heart can also dominate the body's physiological activities through control of the body's mental activities.

the kidney governs the reception of Qi: This implies that the kidney receives the clear air inhaled by the lungs and regulates respiration in order to prevent shallow breathing and to maintain a normal exchange of gases inside and outside the body.

the kidneys govern water: This implies that the kidneys control and regulates water metabolism.

the kidneys store Essence: The kidneys preserve Essence.

the liver and the kidneys share the same origin (Essence and Blood share the same origin): The liver and the kidneys share a common source, the liver Blood and the kidney Essence are inter-generating and inter-transforming, and they come from the essential substances of water and food.

the liver conducts, disperses and ensures the smooth flow of Qi: This function is shown in four aspects.

    a. Promoting the Qi, Blood, and Body Fluid to flow normally

    b. Regulating emotional activities

    c. Aiding digestion and absorption

    d. Promoting menstruation and the discharge of semen

the liver stores Blood: The liver's Blood storage function covers two aspects, storing and regulating Blood.

the lungs govern dispersing and descending: This implies that lung Qi is physiologically characterized by upward and outward dispersion and distribution and downward and inward descending. Dispersing and descending features are the basis of the physiological functions of the lungs.

the lungs govern Qi: The idea means that the entire body's Qi is controlled by the lungs. To be specific, it refers to the lungs dominating the Qi of respiration and dominating the physical Qi of the whole body.

the lungs govern respiration: This idea means that the lungs are the organ responsible for respiratory movement and the place where air coming into and going out of the body is exchanged. The body inhales fresh air and exhales waste gas through the respiratory movement of the lung so as to maintain the normal activities of life. The lungs normalize the metabolic processes of the human body. This activity is known as "getting rid of the stale and taking in the fresh."

the spleen governs blood flow within the vessels: The spleen holds the Blood. This statement describes the role of the spleen in the production of Qi and Blood and its function of preventing extravasation of Blood. Since "Qi contains the Blood," the spleen engenders the Blood and contains it.

the spleen governs transportation and transformation: The spleen dominates transportation and transformation. Transportation and transformation include two aspects, transporting and transforming food, and transporting and transforming water. Transporting and transforming food means that the spleen digests food and assimilates the nutrients. These functions play an important role in the formation of Qi and Blood. The spleen is the source of Qi and Blood and the postnatal base of life. Transporting and transforming water means that the spleen absorbs, disseminates, and excretes water. The spleen plays an important role in regulating and maintaining the balance of water metabolism.

the twelve meridians: The meridians, or "regular meridians," have twelve branches, including the three Yin meridians of the hands and the feet and the three Yang meridians of the hands and the feet. They are the main pathways by which Qi and Blood circulate. The twelve regular meridians originate from and terminate at certain areas and have specific courses and sequences in their circulation. There is also a rule in their distribution in and passing through the trunk and limbs, and they pertain to and connect with the viscera directly in the interior of the body.

The Top Six Groups of Healthy and Anti-Age Plants

TCM prevention before disease onset has two aspects. The first is increasing and maintaining healthy Qi through anti-stress, following a natural rhythm to regulate sleep and activities, eating healthy foods, doing aerobics or relaxed exercises, and applying functional foods or herbal remedies, acupressure, and acupuncture therapies. The second is avoiding invasion by climate factors and applying herbal remedies and vaccines for prevention. There are six groups of functional foods and herbs that can protect one from sickness.

1. Nuts and Seeds

Nuts and seeds are the essence of plants, giving them abundant antioxidants and anti-inflammatory elements. They are rich in nutrients and contain large amounts of protein, trace elements, and vitamins. Regular consumption of nuts and seeds can prevent cardiovascular and cerebrovascular diseases and can make the heart healthier. They can help improve eyesight, prevent senile dementia, provide anti-cancer benefits, and stimulate immunity.

Peanuts are known as a longevity food. Chinese medicine teaches that most nuts and seeds are Neutral or Warm in temperature (walnuts and pine nuts are Warm, while hazelnuts, hemp seeds, peanuts, and cashew nuts are Neutral). They supplement Qi and Blood, strengthen Yin and Yang, moisturize the skin, quench thirst, moisten Dryness, remove annoyance, and reverse Qi reflux. It is suitable for one who has a dry throat and mouth, dry cough, dry or peeling skin, dry itching, and other similar symptoms. Those with excessive Phlegm and congestions or who feel hot and sweaty or those who are Yin-Yang balanced should eat less nuts and seeds or consume with caution. Since most nuts and seeds contain a higher portion of fat, eating too much of them can lead to weight gain, and since they have a high oil content, they are oxidable. It is advisable to consume moderate amounts of nuts and seeds, preferably 20 to 30 grams per day.

2. Fruits

Fruits are rich in beta-carotene and vitamin C, two of the key antioxidants that help form special enzymes and strengthen the body's immunity. In addition, they contain potassium and water-soluble fibers, reduce blood cholesterol levels, and lower the risk of hypertension.

However, fruits are high in sugar and acidic. They should not form as large a part of one's diet as vegetables and grains. Fruits with higher medicinal value that can be applied both as foods and herbs are: Chinese lime, cranberries, apple, mulberries (those are cool), raspberries, pomegranate, schisandra berries, longan fruit, hawthorn (those are Warm), blueberries, blackberries, wolfberries, and fresh jujube (those are Neutral). Many are often used in their dried form (Chinese lime, mulberries, raspberries, schisandra berries, longan fruit, hawthorn, wolfberries, and jujube) and can increase organ functions, stabilize emotions, regulate Yin and Yang, tone Qi, and nourish Blood. Those who experience dizziness, infertility, early onset of aging, and night and frequent urination can choose the way (raw or cooked, fresh or dried) they like to eat fruit. Eat raw and fresh fruits in season or in warm weather, and cooked or dried fruits out of season or in cold weather. When the digestive function is strong, eat raw and fresh fruits, and when it is weak, eat cooked or dried fruits.

The phrase "an apple a day keeps the doctor away" is a folk proverb that emphasizes the apple's comprehensive conditioning capabilities. Eating apples on a regular basis not only inhibits blood cholesterol, but also has a positive impact on blood pressure and improves the intestinal environment. According to the latest research, apples can even affect the lungs, fight pneumonia (antioxidants such as apple polyphenols), and help the lungs rejuvenate.

3. Allium

Allium plants are mostly taken as vegetables and condiments. They are Warm in nature and Spicy in taste, and they can stimulate the body's Qi, Blood, and Yang, increase functions of the kidney, liver, heart, lungs and digestive system, move body Qi and blood circulation, kill viruses and control fungal infection, and open pores and nasal orifices. Garlic, garlic chives, spring onion, onions, and cilantro all contain dietary fiber and organosulfur compounds and are good for probiotics. Among them, garlic chives are the best in early spring.

Oxidized raw garlic has both anti-virus inflammatory and bactericidal functions. Garlic allicin is the compound providing the largest range of garlic's health benefits. Garlic not only can effectively reduce cholesterol, but also prevent high blood pressure and cardiovascular disease and stimulate the body to produce glutathione. Glutathione is the most effective antioxidant in the liver, helping it to detoxify the body and eliminate carcinogens. Those who dislike garlic may prefer garlic leaves and garlic oil.

Chinese medicine teaches that onions have the effects of strengthening the stomach and regulating movement of Qi, detoxifying insect bites, killing insects, and lowering blood lipids. It is commonly used for treating hyperlipidemia, poor appetite, abdominal bloating, trauma, ulcers, and trichomonas vaginitis. Onions contain prostaglandin A, which can reduce peripheral vascular resistance and reduce blood viscosity. They can be used to lower blood pressure, refresh the brain, relieve stress, and prevent colds.

4. Bean Products/Sprouts/Fermented Food

Beans are rich in protein, and as long as they are combined with cereals, they can provide all the amino acids needed by the human body. This includes yellow, black, and green soybeans. Black beans are rich in dietary fiber and antioxidants and have strong antioxidant properties, producing good health effects on the body. Tofu is especially rich in plant-based protein and eating tofu can reduce fat, which is necessary for weight loss. The rich plant protein it contains prevents arteriosclerosis and lowers cholesterol levels. Sprouts contain high levels of concentrated enzymes that make them easier to digest than mature beans. Bean sprouts are rich in antioxidants, which can delay aging.

The active ingredient in tea (green, black, or pu'er), tea polyphenols, is an antioxidant substance. In areas where tea is often consumed, residents have lower rates of cancer, indicating that tea polyphenols can eliminate free radicals and prevent cancer. The anti-oxidation effect of polyphenols can suppress the consumption of vitamin C because it can eliminate active oxygen, inhibiting oxidation. Green tea also removes oil and grease from foods and freshens the breath.

Those who do not like beans or cannot consume many beans because of health conditions can eat more fermented foods like sauerkraut, miso soup, kimchi, yogurt, natto, dried bean sauce, and vinegar. The beneficial bacteria in fermented foods can improve immunity, inhibit chronic inflammation, and support the digestive system. Natto kinase may also soften blood vessels and dissolve thrombi.

5. Whole Grains

Grains, not only the seeds of grasses, can be roughly divided into three categories in China. The first is cereals, including rice (indica, japonica rice, glutinous rice), wheat (wheat, barley, oats, rye), corn, sorghum, millet, yellow rice, and buckwheat. The second category is beans (*shu*), including soybeans, broad beans, peas, mung beans, red beans, kidney beans. The third is potatoes, including sweet potatoes, yam, taro, and cassava. The second category has been listed separately.

Grains contain a large amount of soluble and insoluble fibers, B vitamins, and proteins. They taste mild, are digestible and absorbable, and are an indispensable source of essential nutrients for children and the elderly. Grains can strengthen the spleen and stomach. Properties of grains can be Neutral, Cool, or Warm, making it easy for people to switch between the appropriate grains for winter and summer. For instance, oats and glutinous rice are Warm in temperature, so they can be consumed more in winter. Oats are rich in protein, calcium, riboflavin, and thiamine. They are the only grains in the top tier of antioxidant foods. Daily intake of the right amount of oats can accelerate metabolism, accelerate amino acid synthesis, and promote cell regeneration. Buckwheat contains more protein than rice, wheat, millet, or other grains. The high amount of amino acids contained in buckwheat can also effectively lower cholesterol and control blood sugar. Among the amino acids in buckwheat, flavonoids are good for blood circulation and heart health, and are known as blood supplements. Buckwheat can improve sleep quality. It also contains powerful antioxidants, which can lower blood lipids, enhance blood vessel elasticity, prevent blood clotting, and reduce blood pressure.

Millet is easy to digest, and it can play a role in benefiting the spleen and stomach for elderly people who suffer from stomach ailments. Millet contains amino acids that can inhibit various inflammations, among which tryptophan also aids in sleep and recuperation. When made into porridge, millet has a layer of delicate sticky substance on top, commonly known as rice oil. Chinese medicine teaches that rice oil is extremely rich in nutrients and has the strongest nourishing power. It is often said that "rice oil can substitute for ginseng soup."

6. Algae Foods/Cruciferous Vegetables

Marine algae are spore plants. Marine algae foods include gelidium amansii (agar), laver, kelp, sea cabbage, wakame, etc. Marine algae contains high amounts of minerals such as calcium, iron, sodium, magnesium, phosphorus, and iodine.

Polysaccharides enhance immunity and anti-cancer activity in marine algae. Marine algae is also rich in various enzymes, vitamins, and dietary fiber, which is not only an antioxidant, but also removes human waste.

Spirulina is an ancient lower prokaryotic single-cell or multicellular aquatic plant. It is native to the alkaline lakes in the tropical regions of Chad and Mexico and has long been consumed by local residents. Spirulina is widely distributed in the warm salt and fresh waters of China. It is rich in protein and various amino acids. Spirulina reduces the toxic and side effects of cancer treatments such as radiotherapy and chemotherapy and stabilizes the immune functions. It can lower blood lipids, treat childhood anemia, malnutrition, and physical weakness after illness. Spirulina can be used as health food for body building and weight control and for the elderly, women, and children.

Chinese medicine teaches that seaweed and kelp are Salty in taste, Cold in temperature, and can expel Phlegm, soften hard masses, and regulate liver and kidney energy movements, which are effective for lymphatic tuberculosis and simple iodine deficiency goiters.

Cruciferous vegetables are common vegetables. Due to their higher health value and efficacy, people have gradually begun to pay attention to them. They include bok choy, cabbage, Chinese cabbage, cauliflower, broccoli, shepherd's purse, and radish.

Many traditional Chinese medicines also belong to this family, such as white mustard seeds and radish seeds. Its common effect is prevention of cancer. An epidemiological investigation showed that the consumption of these vegetables was negatively correlated with the incidence of gastric cancer, colon cancer, esophageal cancer, lung cancer, endometrial cancer, and pancreatic cancer. Its active ingredients such as isothiocyanate and indol-3-carbinol have been shown to have anti-cancer effects in research. The Food Nutrition and Oncology Group of the American Cancer Society and the National Security Council have recommended eating more cruciferous vegetables to reduce the incidence of tumors. Cruciferous vegetables contain sulforaphane, which can prevent and treat cancer, and have holistic beauty effects. The flavonoids they contain have a high medicinal value and are used to prevent cardiovascular and cerebrovascular diseases, such as reducing the brittleness of blood vessels, improving the permeability of blood vessels, lowering blood lipids and cholesterol, preventing and treating geriatric hypertension, cerebral hemorrhages, coronary heart disease, angina pectoris, and dilation of coronary blood vessels, and increasing coronary flow. Many flavonoids have antitussive, expectorant, antiasthmatic, and antibacterial functions, while also generating liver protection, detoxification, protection against fungus, and treatment of acute and chronic hepatitis and cirrhosis.

In Chinese herbal medicine, radish seeds are Neutral in temperature, and Sweet and Spicy in taste. White mustard seeds are Hot in temperature, and Spicy in taste. They regulate Phlegm, Qi, and Blood. They can adjust the metabolism of Qi, Blood, and Body Fluids. They can regulate indigestion, fullness of the abdomen, dysuria, constipation, and edema. Shepherd's purse enters the Blood and adjusts digestive and reproductive system hemorrhages, such as vomiting blood, blood in the stool, heavy menstruation, prolonged lochiorrhea, and so on.

Seasonal Foods

Heathy eating includes eating seasonal and local products. Be sure to select seasonal produce in order to get the most nutrients and health benefits. For instance, some fruits that are seasonal in the summer can assist with cooling the body. Due to globalization and technological advancements in agriculture, some food items formerly available only during the summer may now be purchased year-round, but this disrupts the natural rhythms and is not conducive to promoting health. Below are examples of each season's common foods in the northern hemisphere.

Common Foods in Four Seasons			
	Neutral	Cool	Warm
Spring (Mar–May)	Pea, Carrot*, Mushroom, Chinese cabbage	Tomato, Celery, Spinach, Cucumber, White radish, Bamboo shoot	Onion, Parsnip, Water cress, Sward bean, Garlic chive
Summer (June–Aug)	Rice, Grape, Almond, Beetroot, Coconut, Wolfberry, Yellow soybean	Lettuce, Zucchini, Eggplant, Strawberry, Watermelon	Basil, Leek, Squash, Cherry, Raspberry, Long bean
Autumn (Sep–Nov)	Fig, Olive, Corn, Licorice, Peanut, Pumpkin, Hazelnut, Gingko nut, Lotus seed, Sunflower seed	Apple*, Lemon, Tomato, Celery, Grapefruit, Cranberry, Asparagus, Sea vegetables	Peach, Jujube, Sweet potato, Pomegranate, Chestnut, Nuts
Winter (Dec–Feb)	Tangerine, Shiitake mushroom*		Kumquat, Sweet orange

Note:
*Carrot: local harvest available from storage through autumn.
*Apple: cold storage until spring.
*Shiitake mushroom: harvest in winter, spring and autumn.

Three Case Studies in Longevity

Case One: Zhang Jize, born in 1926, now 94 years old, prestigious TCM professor, Board of Director of Menghe Current

Healthy awareness:

• Zhang Jize thinks benevolence (*ren* 忍) and peace (*he* 和) are precious. Traditional philosophies such as Confucianism and Taoism are the spiritual sources that support his teaching, clinical work and preventive healthcare.

• He follows his own rhythm to maintain work-life balance and exercises on a regular basis.

• He is an optimist and able to regulate his own emotions.

State of mind: Zhang Jize is indifferent to fame and fortune and enjoys his daily life. He pours his heart and enthusiasm into medical consultation and passing his family legacy and medical expertise to the next generation of apprentices. His core value is lifelong learning, which lends the credence to the old saying that one is never too old to learn. He always does things that are within his power, including housework.

Diet: Following his TCM body clock, Zhang Jize eats three meals a day to refresh the Yang and Yin energies, eating breakfast at 6:30 to 7:00 am, lunch at 12 noon, and dinner at 6 pm in all four seasons. He drinks warm water on an empty stomach and eats a natural, balanced diet. He eats a variety of foods and stops eating before he is completely full. For breakfast, he eats an egg, five dates, and complex carbohydrates, such as whole grain porridge, oatmeal, glutinous rice, millet, red beans, or smashed corn. For snacks, he rotates on weekly basis among steamed bread (with vegetable, vegetable and meat, red bean paste, sesame stuffing, or steamed open dumplings). For lunch and dinner, he eats three meat and vegetable dishes with one pot of soup. Most dishes are vegetables, and he prefers seafood (such as fish and shrimp) as his meat dish.

Healthy lifestyle: He exercises moderately according to different stages of life. After 70, he exercised within his strength to reduce the strain on joints and muscles. After 80, he took a stroll for 1.5 to 2 hours every day. After 90, he walked for 1.5 hours every day. He would swing his arms as he walked around his house on rainy and snowy days.

In the afternoon, he rests half an hour to one hour a day. When taking a stroll outdoors, he brings foods and daily necessities for home. He soaks his feet with herbal medicine packs to promote blood circulation and remove blood stasis. The packs include safflower and mugwort. He sleeps at 9 pm every day and massages his eyes, ears, and abdomen 100 times before getting up in the morning.

He had practiced in his TCM clinic five mornings a week since he retired (till now) and hand-written 3,000 to 5,000 Chinese characters for prescriptions each day. He is the oldest TCM professor practicing in the Jiangsu Province TCM Hospital (medical staff of 3,000). In his leisure time, he cooks, takes care of the flowers and other plants, practices calligraphy, and pursues academic activities. His friends and family members often ask him to write inscriptions.

Case Two: Deng Tietao (1916–2019), 103 years old, first group of national medical professors, doctoral supervisor

Healthy awareness:

• An ounce of prevention is worth a pound of cure. One should be moral and humane to achieve a stable, peaceful state of mind and to obtain physical and mental harmony and eventually prolong his or her life.

• His preventive healthcare included, according to his physical situation, daily practice of Deng Family Qigong, starting from middle age.

• Following his own rhythm to maintain a work-life balance, he engaged in exercise and entertainment on a regular basis.

State of mind: He followed Confucian ethics, treating all the elderly like his own elderly parents, and treating all children like his own children. He had a balanced exercise-rest rhythm. To maintain a quiet mind, he practiced calligraphy and meditation, combining physical activities to increase energy. He pursued new clinical fields throughout his life and devoted himself to TCM theories and clinical research fields.

Diet: He believed that eating a variety of foods and keeping a moderate diet could harmonize the internal organs and achieve longevity. He followed the classic *Yellow Emperor's Internal Canon of Medicine*, consuming cereal, seeds, meat, and vegetables to supplement energy, Blood, and Essence in order to maintain health. In his daily life, he emphasized that the regulation of digestive functions was not only important for curing sickness to save the patient, but was also applicable to his daily preventive healthcare. He believed that failure to take meals on time or being either hungry or full for too long would harm the system and might impact one's health.

He followed his TCM body clock, eating three meals a day, with breakfast at 8:30 am. He drank a cup of milk a day, stopping his meals before he was completely full. Before lunch, at around 11 am he drank a small cup of hot tea, then ate lunch at 12 pm and dinner at 6 pm. He preferred to eat digestible, mild flavored foods. He ate rice as a staple food, accompanied with a portion of potato, pumpkin, oatmeal, buckwheat, beans, fish and shrimp, and egg and milk, and he ate red dates and walnuts as supplements to maintain a balanced diet, using radish, pear, dragon fruit, and vegetables to reduce Deficiency of Fire.

Healthy lifestyle: After his mid-90s, Deng Tietao got up at 7 am and drank a cup of warm water. After that, he combed his scalp with both hands (taking turns, 100 times per hand) and practiced Qigong on the balcony, since the average temperature in Guangzhou is over 20°C.

After breakfast, he read the paper and magazines or composed articles and practiced calligraphy. After lunch, he read books or newspapers and took a 2-hour nap at 1:30 pm. If the weather allowed, he would go downstairs to take a stroll and absorb some sunshine. After he returned home, he would practice standing Qigong for 20 minutes if he was energetic enough, and massage the Zusanli (ST 36) and Yongquan points (KI 1) for another 20 minutes. After dinner, he watched the news on TV. He would soak his feet in a herbal medicine decoction or hot water and massage his toes, pelma, and ankles to promote blood circulation, relieve tiredness, and strengthen his body.

When Deng Tietao turned 101, he was still healthy, clear minded, could express himself smoothly, had good eyesight and hearing, and could walk steadily.

Case Three: Zheng Ji (1900–2010), lived until 110, well-known biochemist, nutritionist, and educationist

Healthy awareness:

• He pursued preventive healthcare. With less desire and compulsion, he was always at ease and comfortable. He worked and rested moderately and took care of his diets. He visited a doctor as soon as he suffered from any indisposition and was not overly anxious even when seriously ill. He took things as they came, and constantly strove to become stronger. He advocated the theory that man is an integral part of nature, so he pursued natural life span.

• He lived, ate, worked and exercised in a self-disciplinary way.

• He lived in harmony with the nature and kept an eye on nutritional information and listened to his body.

State of mind: He believed nothing would be too complicated if it was not taken too seriously, so to obtain a healthy body, one should remain calm. He never treated himself as an old man, but could endure hardship and take on responsibilities. In his opinion, this mainly depended on his own condition. He devoted his whole heart to science, did not think too much about his age, and did not admit to being old.

Diet: He followed modern nutrition science and ate a scientific diet, followed natural rhythms, and balanced meat and vegetable portions, taking larger proportions of vegetable. He only ate vegetable oil and avoided eating grease or fat, only occasionally eating deep-fried, preserved, and overly spicy, salty, or sweet foods. He followed his TCM body clock and ate 3 meals a day, eating 20 percent less and chewing food well before swallowing.

He believed that people over 90 should always eat a highly digestible, low fat, low calorie, low sugar, vitamin rich diet with plenty of dietary fiber.

For breakfast and dinner, he had a cup of milk, 2 organic eggs, a bowl of jujube soup (5 pieces of jujube, 3 pieces of longan, 15 to 20 pieces of wolfberries), and a piece of steamed bread (replaceable by noodles, wonton, or porridge). He also ate porridge, chives with fried eggs, and lotus root starch with steamed red bean bread for dinner. His butler said that he would not eat a meal without milk, porridge, and lotus root starch and an appropriate amount of Vitamin A, B, C, and E, which he estimated as 1 pill of VA, 2 pills of VB1 (10 mg/pill), 2 pills of VB2 (5 mg/pill), VC (300 — 600 mg), VE (50 — 100 mg).

He divided the pills into two portions each day.

Healthy lifestyle: In his early years, he devoted most of his enthusiasm into absorbing knowledge and carving out his career in biochemistry and nutrition science. He also loves physical activity. When he was in his 50s, he began gardening, trying to cultivate vegetables, flowers, and trees. In his 60s, he paid extra attention to physical exercises, and in his 70s, he turned to acquisition of aging and anti-aging knowledge. He also developed a hobby of reading ancient Chinese poetry, especially from the Tang and Song dynasties. He also wrote some poetry to entertain himself and appreciated traditional Chinese painting. Since he was also interested in traveling, he planned biannual trips (during summer and winter vocation). After he turned 100, Professor Zhen was still energetic, quick-witted, and fit as a fiddle, compiling a biochemistry history of China.

He followed a regular sleep-wake rhythm, getting up at 6 am and massaging himself from scalp to toe for a quarter hour to 20 minutes before getting up. After freshening up, he took another 15 to 20 minutes for Qigong exercises, which included warm-up activities, upper body movements, lower limb movements, and stretching exercises to stimulate body metabolism. After lunch, he would take a one or two hours' nap at 12:45. When he was tired, caught a cold, or uncomfortable, he would rest in bed, a habit he persisted in for decades.

Professor Zhen offered a conclusion summarizing his preventive healthcare tips:

Be open-minded, and establish positive, stable emotional health.

Maintain a regular sleep-wake rhythm and rest-exercise rhythm.

Pay attention to dietetic and environmental hygiene and embrace the natural environment, fresh air, and sunshine.

Eat in moderation, drink less liquor, do not smoke, control sexual desire, and abandon bad habits.

Last but not least, take precautions to prevent accidental injuries, and never overlook indispositions.

The Categorization of Prescriptions According to the Specific Function of Chinese Medical Herbs

In the Chinese materia medica, there are exterior-releasing pungent-warm herbs, such as cinnamon sticks. For prescriptions, there are corresponding exterior-releasing pungent-warm formulas, such as a cinnamon stick decoction, which is made up of five kinds of herbs. The other types of materia medica and corresponding prescriptions are similar. The following table offers more examples of prescription categorizations. You may also refer to Chapter Two of Part Three for more information regarding Chinese materia medica and prescriptions.

The Chinese Materia Medica	Examples	TCM Prescriptions	Examples
Exterior-releasing: Pungent-Warm	Cinnamon stick	Exterior-releasing Pungent-Warm formulas	Cinnamon stick decoction 桂枝汤
Exterior-releasing: Pungent-Cool	Mulberry leaf	Exterior-releasing Pungent-Cool formulas	Mulberry leaf & chrysanthemum beverage 桑菊饮
Heat-clearing	Gardenia	Heat-clearing formulas	Gardenia & black bean sauce decoction 栀子豉汤
Downward-draining	Peach kernel	Downward-draining formulas	Five kernels pill 五仁丸
Wind-damp-dispelling	Mulberry stick	Wind-damp-dispelling formulas	Pubescent angelica and mistletoe decoction 独活寄生汤
Dampness-transforming	Eupatorium	Dampness-transforming formulas	Agastache Qi-correcting powder 藿香正气散
Promoting the movement of water and percolating Dampness	Pearl barley, poria	Promoting the movement of water and percolating Dampness formulas	Poria pill 茯苓丸
Interior-warming	Sichuan pepper, dried ginger	Interior-warming formulas	Center-regulating pill 理中丸
Qi-regulating	Tangerine peel and leaf	Qi-regulating formulas	Tangerine peel and bamboo shavings decoction 橘皮竹茹汤

Stopping bleeding	Cacumen biotae, lotus rhizome node	Stopping bleeding formulas	Ten charred substances powder 十灰散
Blood-quickening and stasis-dispelling	Safflower and saffron, peach kernel	Blood-quickening and stasis-dispelling formulas	Peach kernel and carthamus four substances decoction 桃红四物汤
Food-dispersing	Hawthorn berry, redish seed	Food-dispersing formulas	Harmony-preserving pill 保和丸
Transforming Phlegm	Mustard seed	Transforming Phlegm formulas	Three-seed filial devotion decoction 三子养亲汤
Stopping coughing and calming wheezing	Almond, loquat leaf	Stopping coughing and calming wheezing formulas	Arrest wheezing decoction 定喘汤
Spirit-quieting	Radix polygalae, Chinese arborvitae seed	Spirit-quieting formulas	Celestial emperor heart-supplementing elixir 天王补心丹
Calming the liver and expelling Wind	Cassia seed	Calming the liver and expelling Wind formulas	Gastrodia and uncaria decoction 天麻钩藤饮
Supplementing: Qi-supplementing	Astragalus, Chinese yam	Qi-supplementing formulas	Center-supplementing and Qi-boosting decoction 补中益气汤
Supplementing: Blood-nourishing	Angelica, longan fruit	Supplementing and Blood-nourishing formulas	Four substances decoction 四物汤
Supplementing: Yin-enriching	wolfberry, lily bulb	Supplementing and Yin-enriching formulas	Lily bulb metal-securing decoction 百合固金汤
Supplementing: Yang-fortifying	Walnut, fructus psoraleae	Supplementing and Yang-fortifying formulas	Right-restoring pill 右归丸
Securing and stringing	Schisandra berry, lotus seed	Securing and stringing formulas	Golden lock Essence-securing pill 金锁固精丸
Orifice-opening	Acorus	Orifice-opening formulas	Peaceful palace bovine bezoar pill 安宫牛黄丸

Self-Help Meridian Points and Their Locations

In the following table, all points mentioned in this book are listed with an explanation of their locations. You can also locate them by referring to the meridian maps on pages 122–126.

Point Name	Number	Location
Anmian	EX-HN 16	At the middle point of the depression behind the ear next to the ear lobe and the Fengchi point (GB 20).
Baihui	GV 20	On the middle line of the head, at the cross section of the line running from the nose to the base of the head and both ears, at the top of the head.
Chize	LU 5	Bend the elbow, on the crease, in the depression on the radial side of the tendon.
Cuanzhu	BL 2	On the head, in the depression at the medial end of the eyebrow.
Daling	PC 7	Between two tendons at the midpoint of the wrist and palm transverse crease.
Dannang	EX-LE 6	On the lower leg, 1 cun inferior to the Yanglingquan point (GB 34).
Danzhong	CV 17	Parallel with the intercostal space of the 4th rib, at the front central line.
Dazhu	BL 11	On the upper back, level with the inferior border of the spinous process of the first thoracic vertebra, 1.5 cun lateral to the midline.
Dazhui	GV 14	On the upper back, inferior to the spinous process of the 7th cervical vertebra.
Feishu	BL 13	On the upper back, level with the inferior border of the spinous process of the 3rd thoracic vertebra, 1.5 cun lateral to the midline.
Fengchi	GB 20	On the posterior aspect of the neck, below the occipital bone, on the hairline in a depression on the outer area of the largest tendon (on both right and left sides).
Fengfu	GV 16	On the posterior aspect of the neck, immediately inferior to the occipital bone on the midline.
Ganshu	BL 18	On the back, level with the inferior border of the spinous process of the 9th thoracic vertebra, 1.5 cun lateral to the midline.

Geshu	BL 17	On the back, level with the inferior border of the spinous process of the 7th thoracic vertebra, 1.5 cun lateral to the midline.
Guanyuan	CV 4	On the midline of the abdomen, 3 cun below the umbilicus.
Hegu	LI 4	On the fleshy part of the hand between the thumb and forefinger. Using your left hand, match the first crease of the thumb joint to the edge of the middle fleshy portion of the right hand and pressing down on the thumb. Meet the forefinger of the left hand on the opposite side and press.
Houxi	SI 3	On the little finger side of the palmar, proximal to the head of the 5th bone, at the border of the red & white flesh.
Jianjing	GB 21	On the superior aspect of the shoulder, midway between the 7th cervical vertebra and the high point of the acromioclavicular articulation.
Jianliao	TE 14	At the posterior aspect of the shoulder joint, immediately posterior and inferior to the acromion.
Jianyu	LI 15	On the lateral aspect of the shoulder, inferior to the acromioclavicular articulation, between the anterior and medial portions of the deltoid muscle, anterior of the depressions that form when the arm abducted.
Jianzhen	SI 9	On the posterior aspect of the upper arm, 1 cun directly above the back of the armpit fold.
Jingmen	GB 25	On the lower back, at the inferior border of the tip of the 12th rib.
Lanwei	EX-LE 7	On the anterior aspect of the lower leg, at the most sensitive site along the Stomach Meridian in the area about 2 cun below Zusanli point (ST 36).
Liangqiu	ST 34	On the anterior aspect of the thigh, 2 cun proximal to the super lateral corner of the patella, on the line connecting the anterior superior iliac spine and the lateral border of the patella.
Lieque	LU 7	1.5 cun proximal to the wrist, in a crevice on the lateral edge of the radius just proximal to the styloid process.
Neiguan	PC 6	Between two tendons, 2 cun over the wrist transverse crease.
Pishu	BL 20	On the back, level with the inferior border of the spinous process of the 11th thoracic vertebra, 1.5 cun lateral to the midline.

Qihai	CV 6	On the lower abdomen, 1.5 cun inferior to the umbilicus on the midline.
Qimen	LR 14	At the 6th rib under the nipple.
Quchi	LI 11	On the lateral aspect of the elbow, in the depression at the lateral end of the crease just distal to the lateral epicondyle of the humerus.
Sanyinjiao	SP 6	On the rear edge of the shinbone, 3 cun above the ankle.
Shaohai	HT 3	At the bend of the elbow, at the medial end of the cubital crease, in the depression just anterior to the medial epicondyle of the humerus.
Shenmen	HT 7	Between the first and second line of the wrist in the depression at the upper forearm to the small finger side of the hand, inside the wrist crease of the large tendon.
Shenshu	BL 23	On the lower back, level with the inferior border of the spine process of the two lumbar vertebra, 1.5 cun lateral of the midline.
Shixuan	EX-UE 11	On the tips of the ten fingers, a few millimeters from the nail.
Shuifen	CV 9	On the upper abdomen, 1 cun superior to the umbilicus on the midline.
Shuigou	GV 26	Above the upper lip, in the crease, one third of the distance from the base of the nasal septum to the center of the red skin on the upper lip.
Sibai	ST 2	In the depression of the orifice under the eye socket, under the central line of the eyeball.
Taichong	LR 3	On the dorsal aspect of the foot, in the depression distal to the junction of the first and second metatarsal bones.
Taixi	KI 3	At the ankle joint, midway between the tip of the inside ankle and tendon.
Taiyang	EX-HN 5	In the depression about 1 cun behind the space between the outer tip of the brow and outer eye corner.
Taiyuan	LU 9	On the palmar aspect of the wrist, in the depression at the radial end of the wrist crease, between the artery and tendon.
Tianshu	ST 25	On the abdomen, level with the center of the umbilicus, 2 cun lateral to the midline.
Waiguan	TE 5	On the palmar side of the forearm, 2 cun proximal above the wrist, midway between the two bones.
Weishu	BL 21	On the back, level with the inferior border of the spinous process of the 12th thoracic vertebra, 1.5 cun lateral to the midline.

Xingjian	LR 2	On the dorsal aspect of the foot, on the web area between the first and second toe at the line coloration of white and pink skin.
Xinshu	BL 15	On the upper back, level with the inferior border of the spinous process of the 5th thoracic vertebra, 1.5 cun lateral to the midline.
Xuanzhong	GB 39	3 cun above the tip of outside ankle.
Xuehai	SP 10	(1) When the knee is flexed, the point is 2 cun above the medial superior border of the patella on the bulge of the medial portion of quadriceps femoris. (2) When the knee is flexed, cup your right palm to the patient's left knee, with the thumb on the medial side and other 4 fingers directed proximally and the thumb forming an angle of 45 degrees with the index finger. The point is where the tip of your thumb rests.
Yanglingquan	GB 34	On the lateral aspect of the lower leg in the depression below the head of the fibula.
Yifeng	TE 17	Underneath the earlobe, in the hollow between the mandible and the mastoid process.
Yinbai	SP 1	0.1 cun below the base of the nail on the medial side of the big toe.
Yintang	GV 29	Between the eyebrows, equidistant between them.
Yingxiang	LI 20	0.5 cun beside the wing of nose, in the nasolabial groove.
Yinlingquan	SP 9	In the depression on the inner edge of the shinbone by the knee.
Yongquan	KI 1	At the junction of the anterior third and posterior two thirds of the sole, in the deepest depression when the foot is in plantor flexion.
Zhangmen	LR 13	On the lateral aspect of the abdomen, approximately on the midaxillary line, immediately below the tip of the 11th rib.
Zhigou	TE 6	On the palmar side of the forearm, 3 cun proximal above the wrist, midway between the two bones.
Zhiyin	BL 67	0.1 cun below the base of the nail on the lateral aspect of the little toe.
Zhongwan	CV 12	On the upper abdomen, on the middle line, two finger-width below the chest bone, in the depression.
Zusanli	ST 36	On the anterior aspect of the lower leg, 3 cun inferior to Dubi point (ST 35), about one finger-width lateral to the tibia.

Comprehensive Methods for Preventing Influenza

Influenza is a commonly encountered, serious epidemic disease. Combining modern and traditional Chinese medicine may assist in helping to reduce morbidity and to diminish the severity of the illness, while TCM may further play a role in its prevention.

Early in the year 2000, an influenza virus of the Sydney A type spread from England over the whole of Europe and the USA. Millions of people fell ill and several thousand people died. Approximately 14 countries suffered this epidemic, 12 in Europe and 2 in Asia.

Historically we can observe that people suffer epidemics of influenza somewhere in the world every year. The last serious influenza epidemic in the UK was from 1989 to 1990. The infection rate was very high (600 out of every 10,000) and 26,000 people in all died from that single epidemic. Although the precise total is not known, the morbidity rate was higher in the winter of 1999 to 2000 (7% to 20% in Europe and the USA), especially among the elderly, although the mortality rate was lower.

In the USA, influenza combined with pneumonia is the "fifth killer" of humans after heart disease, cancer, stroke and pulmonary emphysema.

Fatal influenza is frequently epidemic in Europe and the USA but rarer in Asia. This is because people have different reactions to influenza according to geographical location. Influenza tends to affect the lung and the heart lightly in Asia, but more seriously in Europe where the central nervous system is also more likely to be affected. Examples of nervous system sequelae include post viral syndromes manifesting with such symptoms as high or low fever, heavy headedness or dull headache, lack of concentration or depression, etc. This geographical variation may result from different body constitution and environments among different races.

Influenza is not only the cause of sudden high morbidity, but is also influential in the cause of many chronic diseases, for example pneumonia, bronchitis and chronic fatigue syndrome. Therefore, as well as improving health education, multiple effective measures should be used to control the spread of the virus in order to save lives and money.

As a type of acute respiratory tract infection, influenza can reach epidemic proportions very quickly. Prevention is therefore more important than treatment. People can take a few steps to assist in prevention, for example:

• Avoid crowded spaces and maintain good ventilation in all rooms.

• Use vinegar as a simple method of sterilization to fumigate a room, or use 10% water-soluble vinegar as nasal drops.

• Acupuncture or moxibustion as prevention: on the points of Zusanli (ST 36), Yongquan (KI 1), Qihai (CV 6), Guanyuan (CV 4). Treat daily for three successive days. This can strengthen the spleen and kidney energy to improve the body's immune reaction.

• Herbs: The aim is to clear Heat and toxicity by promoting diuresis, improve superficial immunity and eliminates Dampness. This will restrict the effect of the virus and reduce Heat: Ban Lan Gen (Radix Isatidis seu Baphicacanthi) 15 g, Da Qing Ye (Folium Daqingye) 15 g, Guan Zhong (Rhizoma Cyrtomii Fortunei) 10 g, Jin Yin Hua (Flos Lonicerae Japonicae) 10 g, Pu Gong Ying (Herba Taraxaci Mongolici cum Radice) 10 g, Qiang Huo (Rhizoma et Radix Notopterygii) 10 g, Huo Xiang (Herba Agastaches seu Pogostemi) 10 g, Pei Lan (Herba Eupatorii Fortunei) 10 g, Ge Gen (Radix Puerariae) 10 g, Hua Shi (Talcum) 5 g, Sheng Gan Cao (Radix Glycyrrhizae Uralensis) 3 g. Choose 3 to 6 of these herbs and prepare as a decoction. Dosage: twice a day, 5 to 7 days as a course.

• Foods that increase resistance to influenza:

Cold condition: before and during epidemics regularly consume leek, spring onion, garlic, onion, caper, walnut, date, sweet potato.

Hot condition: before and during epidemics regularly consume artichoke, radish, dandelion leaf, chicory, mint, towel gourd, mung bean sprout, pear, grapefruit, lemon, orange, water chestnut, momordica fruit (fructus momordicae grosvenori), seed of great burdock, pomegranate.

All conditions: before and during epidemics regularly consume olive, loquat, apricot, almonds, fig, Chinese yam, black fungus.

• Exercises including Tai Chi, Qigong, walking and slow running help to strengthen Defensive Qi and develop immunity from disease.

Index

A

acupressure 8, 10, 15, 27, 39, 40,
    42–44, 50, 99, 109, 127, 128,
    148, 161, 261, 269
acupuncture 8, 10–12, 15–18, 24,
    25, 50, 99, 101, 109–112, 114,
    115, 117, 127, 133–140, 142, 143,
    148, 149, 154, 157, 158, 160,
    161, 163, 253, 254, 269, 288
Anmian point 125, 128, 129, 283
anti-aging 7, 23, 177, 225, 280
anti-bacterial 173
anti-cancer 177, 269, 273, 274
anti-diuretic 181
anti-hormonal 174
anti-inflammatory 181, 269
anti-oxidant 175, 179
anti-radiation 179
anti-tumor 179, 181
Ashi point 115, 128, 156, 163

B

Ba Duan Jin 13, 18, 208, 230–233
Baihui point 44, 126, 127, 129, 258,
    261, 283
balance 9, 10, 12, 15, 18, 21, 23,
    25–27, 31, 35, 39, 43, 50, 51, 59,
    60, 62–64, 66–68, 73, 74, 82, 83,
    87, 89, 91, 105, 109, 110, 112,
    117, 134, 136, 139, 143, 148,
    155, 167–169, 172, 200, 202,
    207, 211, 219, 221, 224–227,
    229, 230, 233, 234, 237, 240,
    241, 243–245, 250, 255, 256,
    258, 259, 263, 268, 269, 276–279
Basic Questions 12, 22, 85, 109, 208
beauty 197, 220, 274
breath 12, 13, 15, 24, 43, 47, 48,
    50, 52, 54, 55, 58, 72, 79, 81, 82,
    92, 96, 97, 107, 112, 113, 119,
    122, 131, 149, 174, 175, 178,
    179, 181, 183, 184, 206–214,
    220–224, 231–233, 238, 246,
    252, 266, 272

C

*Categorized Patterns with Clear-Cut
    Treatments* 208
Chinese Pharmacopoeia 188
Chize point 112, 122, 283
Conception Vessel 120, 126, 128,
    262, 266
Confucius 254
Cuanzhu point 150, 283
cupping 11, 12, 15, 50, 110, 111,
    114, 117, 134, 153–161, 163, 246

D

Daling point 123, 128, 283
Dannang point 115, 125, 283
dantian 207, 222
Danzhong point 39, 52, 53, 126,
    133, 264, 283
Dazhu point 125, 133, 283
Dazhui point 110, 126, 151, 152,
    155, 262, 283
dehumidification 154
detoxification 33–35, 58, 62, 64,
    119, 157–159, 178, 190, 192–
    195, 200, 202, 204, 206, 240,
    246, 257, 271, 273, 274, 288
diagnosis 12, 16, 24, 25, 29, 39, 42,
    75, 91, 92, 99, 102, 105, 111,
    112, 114, 115, 118, 119, 148,
    212, 220, 251
Dubi point 124, 130, 286

E

emotion   15, 31, 37–42, 44, 50, 55, 56, 60, 63, 66, 74, 82–86, 91, 167, 184, 232, 237, 240, 244, 245, 247, 248, 254–258, 263, 267, 270, 276, 280
Encyclopedia of Chinese Medicinal Formulas   199

F

Feishu point   110, 125, 155, 283
Fengchi point   40, 113, 125, 129, 151, 155, 249, 283
Fengfu point   126, 249, 283
Fifty-Two Diseases   154
formula   27, 99, 143, 185, 191, 193, 197–204, 281, 282
Formulas for Universal Relief   199
fu   31, 37, 38, 44, 45, 50, 59, 64, 120, 132, 137, 243, 246

G

Ganshu point   115, 125, 283
Geshu point   125, 133, 284
Golden Mirror of the Medical Tradition   154
Gong Yanxian   259
Governing Vessel   120, 126, 163, 236, 262, 266
Great Dictionary of Chinese Herbal Medicine   188
Gua Sha   50, 110, 111, 117, 159–165, 246, 261
Guanyuan point   44, 126, 130, 258, 262, 284, 288

H

Health Quotient   9, 19
Hegu point   42, 122, 128, 140, 163, 262, 284
Houxi point   123, 131, 284

Hua Tuo   224

I

Illustrated Classic of Acupoints on the Bronze Figure   136
Important Formulas Worth a Thousand Gold Pieces   143, 149
improve immunity   143, 183, 216, 269, 270, 272, 273, 288

J

Jianjing point   113, 125, 140, 284
Jianliao point   123, 138, 155, 284
Jianyu point   122, 138, 155, 284
Jianzhen point   123, 130, 155, 284
Jingmen point   125, 262, 284
Jueyin Liver Meridian of the Foot   41, 50, 51, 65, 100, 115, 121, 125, 195
Jueyin Pericardium Meridian of the Hand   65, 100, 121, 123, 148

L

Lanwei point   115, 124, 284
Li Shizhen   187
Liangqiu point   115, 124, 284
Lieque point   43, 112, 122, 130, 284
Lin Peiqin   208
longevity   8, 23, 24, 68, 87, 89, 167, 173, 183, 197, 210, 213, 222, 225, 254, 260, 269, 276, 277
lubricating the skin   197

M

meditation   13, 24, 54, 94, 167, 209, 213, 214, 220–223, 277
moxa   113, 141–146
moxibustion   12, 16, 101, 109–111, 114, 117, 134–136, 138, 140–147, 154, 160, 161, 246, 262, 288

N

needle 18, 102, 109, 127, 134, 135, 137–140, 143, 149, 150, 158, 159

Neiguan point 39, 123, 127, 131, 138, 139, 284

P

pain relief 135, 260

Pishu point 125, 152, 284

pregnancy 62, 66, 134, 140, 144, 159, 165, 194, 264

prescription 11, 12, 17, 39, 40, 42–44, 142, 149, 184, 189, 193, 196–200, 202, 205, 207, 277, 281

Q

Qigong 8, 10, 15, 16, 27, 50, 54, 94, 117, 120, 121, 208, 213, 222, 224, 230–232, 248, 256, 277, 278, 280, 288

Qihai point 126, 258, 285, 288

Qimen point 115, 125, 285

Quchi point 122, 163, 262, 285

R

rehabilitation/recuperation 9, 13, 16, 39, 149, 181, 232, 260, 273

S

Sanyinjiao point 40, 124, 131, 140, 262, 285

Shaohai point 124, 129, 285

Shaoyang Gallbladder Meridian of the Foot 41, 50, 63, 65, 100, 113, 117, 121, 125, 163

Shaoyang *Sanjiao* (Triple Energizer) Meridian of the Hand 65, 100, 121, 123, 145, 148

Shaoyin Heart Meridian of the Hand 39, 65, 100, 121, 124

Shaoyin Kidney Meridian of the Foot 44, 50, 65, 88, 100, 118, 121, 126, 146, 261

Shen Nong's Classic of Materia Medica 187

Shenmen point 40, 124, 129, 261, 285

Shenshu point 44, 125, 131, 152, 262, 285

Shixuan point 11, 124, 128, 163, 285

Shuifen point 126, 262, 285

Shuigou point 11, 126, 128, 163, 285

Sibai point 124, 130, 150, 285

Sun Simiao 143, 149, 259

T

Tai Chi 13, 18, 24, 208, 223–226, 230, 288

Tai Chi Martial Art Theory 224

Taichong point 125, 130, 262, 285

Taixi point 43, 126, 131, 262, 285

Taiyang Bladder Meridian of the Foot 44, 65, 100, 121, 125, 144, 152, 155, 164, 236, 262

Taiyang point 124, 150, 151, 285

Taiyang Small Intestine Meridian of the Hand 31, 39, 65, 100, 121, 123

Taiyin Lung Meridian of the Hand 43, 45, 65, 100, 112, 117, 121, 122

Taiyin Spleen Meridian of the Foot 41, 65, 100, 117, 121, 124, 145, 262

Taiyuan point 43, 122, 133, 285

The Grand Compendium of Materia Medica 187

The Spiritual Pivot 12, 135

The Systematic Classic of Acupuncture and Moxibustion 135

Tianshu point 42, 124, 131, 285
Treatise on Cold Damage 116, 149, 199, 200, 201
Treatise on Exogenous Febrile Disease 142
Tuina 12, 15–17, 50, 109–111, 136, 147–149, 152, 163

W

Waiguan point 123, 132, 155, 285
Wang Zongyue 224
weight loss 93, 154, 172, 231, 252, 271
Weishu point 115, 125, 285
Wu Qian 154

X

Xingjian point 39, 125, 129, 286
Xinshu point 125, 152, 286
Xuanzhong point 125, 132, 262, 286
Xuehai point 124, 131, 286

Y

Yang 12, 20–27, 29, 30, 32, 33, 39, 41, 43, 44, 52, 55, 56, 60, 64, 65, 67, 68, 73, 77–83, 85, 86, 88, 90, 93, 95–97, 99, 102, 104–106, 117, 120–122, 132, 136, 139, 140, 142, 145, 149, 157, 163, 168, 169, 172, 188, 189, 194, 196, 197, 200, 201, 203, 204, 211, 218, 219, 221, 224, 227, 229, 230, 233, 234, 239, 240–250, 255, 263, 268–270, 276, 282
Yanglingquan point 101, 115, 125, 132, 283, 286
Yangming Large Intestine Meridian of the Hand 43, 45, 65, 88, 100, 121, 122, 163
Yangming Stomach Meridian of the Foot 41, 65, 66, 89, 100, 114, 117, 118, 120, 121, 124, 147, 189, 284
Yellow Emperor's Internal Canon of Medicine 11, 109, 135, 142, 149, 159, 199, 233, 240, 241, 245, 251, 259, 277
Yifeng point 123, 249, 286
Yin 12, 20–27, 29, 30, 32, 34, 35, 39, 41, 43, 44, 55, 56, 64–68, 73, 78–84, 88, 93, 96, 97, 99, 102, 104–106, 117, 120–122, 132, 136, 139, 149, 157, 168, 169, 181, 183, 196, 197, 200, 201, 203, 205, 206, 211, 219–221, 224, 227, 230, 233, 234, 239–242, 244, 247–250, 262, 263, 268–270, 276, 282
Yinbai point 124, 145, 286
Yingxiang point 122, 130, 286
Yinlingquan point 124, 262, 286
Yintang point 126, 128, 286
Yongquan point 114, 126, 130, 146, 278, 286, 288

Z

zang 31, 37, 38, 44, 45, 50, 59, 64, 120, 132, 243
Zhang Zhongjing 116, 149, 199
Zhang Zihe 27
Zhangmen point 125, 132, 286
Zhigou point 123, 131, 286
Zhiyin point 125, 144, 286
Zhongwan point 126, 132, 144, 286
Zusanli point 42, 101, 113, 115, 124, 127, 130, 142, 258, 262, 278, 284, 286, 288